THE AFTERWORLD

THE AFTERWORLD

Long Covid and International Relations

Edited by Frédéric Mérand and Jennifer Welsh

University of Ottawa Press
2024

Les Presses de l'Université d'Ottawa
University of Ottawa Press

The University of Ottawa Press (UOP) is proud to be the oldest of the francophone university presses in Canada and the oldest bilingual university publisher in North America. Since 1936, UOP has been enriching intellectual and cultural discourse by producing peer-reviewed and award-winning books in the humanities and social sciences, in French and in English.

www.Press.uOttawa.ca

Library and Archives Canada Cataloguing in Publication

Title: The afterworld : long COVID and international relations / edited by Frédéric Mérand and Jennifer Welsh.
Other titles: Afterworld (Ottawa, Ont.)
Names: Mérand, Frédéric, 1976- editor. | Welsh, Jennifer M. (Jennifer Mary), 1965- editor.
Series: Health and society (University of Ottawa Press)
Description: Series statement: Health and society | Includes bibliographical references.
Identifiers: Canadiana (print) 20240292863 | Canadiana (ebook) 2024029288X | ISBN 9780776641478 (softcover) | ISBN 9780776641553 (hardcover) | ISBN 9780776641485 (PDF) | ISBN 9780776641492 (EPUB)
Subjects: LCSH: International relations. | LCSH: COVID-19 Pandemic, 2020-—Influence.
Classification: LCC JZ1242.A38 2024 | DDC 327—dc23

Legal Deposit: Second Quarter 2024
Library and Archives Canada

Production Team

Copy-editing	Jonathan Dore and Tanina Drvar
Proofreading	Valentina D'Aliesio and Céline Parent
Typesetting	Édiscript enr.
Cover design	Benoit Deneault

Cover Image
Creative Minimalist Hand Painted Abstract Art Stock Vector, Shutterstock, 1936225114

SSHRC ≡ CRSH This book was published with the help of a grant from the Canadian Federation for the Humanities and Social Sciences, through the Awards to Scholarly Publications Program, using funds provided by the Social Sciences and Humanities Research Council of Canada.

The University of Ottawa Press gratefully acknowledges the support extended to its publishing list by the Government of Canada, the Canada Council for the Arts, the Ontario Arts Council, the Social Sciences and Humanities Research Council and the Canadian Federation for the Humanities and Social Sciences through the Scholarly Book Awards (ASPP), and by the University of Ottawa.

Table of Contents

Foreword

Louise Fréchette
Former Deputy Secretary-General of the United Nations

When asked about his assessment of the French Revolution, Deng Xiaoping reportedly replied, "It's too early to tell." Of course, only time can accurately assess the lasting impacts of a crisis.

We heard since the start of the pandemic that "the world will never be the same again," but how might the COVID-19 pandemic bring about sweeping changes to our daily lives, our collective life, and relations between countries? The researchers in this book take an informed, objective look at the various dimensions of the pandemic. Their analysis of its impact on the economy, health care, international security, and many other issues helps us to see more clearly, to distinguish the longer-lasting effects from those that are likely to be short-lived, and to place them in the broader context of existing societal trends.

The emergence of COVID-19 has highlighted—more clearly than ever before—the weaknesses and failings of both national and international systems in preventing and managing health crises. It has also brought to light the harsh reality of vulnerable or marginalized groups for whom existing social safety nets have proved inadequate. It has further widened the gap between rich and poor countries. The analyses contained in this volume offer a detailed map of the grey areas the pandemic exposed and identify a range of measures that could be implemented to avoid history repeating itself when the next pandemic—because there will be one—arrives on our doorstep.

In several countries, corrective measures were taken in light of the experience gained during the first waves of the pandemic. For example, in Canada, improvements were made to how retirement homes are managed, and to increase medical supply stocks. Think, too, of the telework boom, to which both the private and public sectors adapted remarkably well. The significant—and unprecedented—action governments have taken to counter the economic effects of the pandemic may pave the way for a new kind of economic and fiscal policy.

It would have been satisfying to see an equally innovative spirit in international cooperation. Unfortunately, the opposite was true. Tensions between the United States and China are spilling over into the World Health Organization (WHO), where the controversy surrounding the origin of the virus is mobilizing minds and undermining the organization's credibility. It is hard to imagine a day when the WHO will be granted the powers and resources it needs to fulfill its vital mandate of research, advice, and coordination. This geostrategic dynamic also risks fuelling protectionist tendencies in the name of safeguarding supply and self-sufficiency. Developing countries—for whom international trade and supply chain contribution are a key driver of economic growth—risk paying the price for production capacity being repatriated to developed countries.

And what about the global management of vaccines—or lack thereof? China cannot be blamed for the vaccine race that has allowed the richest countries to monopolize vaccine acquisition for the benefit of their own populations, leaving the rest of the planet unprotected. It was almost obscene to talk about a fifth dose when billions of people were still waiting for their first. What made this situation all the more disturbing was that all experts are in agreement that more dangerous variants can emerge in unvaccinated populations. It was not especially surprising that governments turned a deaf ear to calls for human solidarity, but it was harder to understand why they were so indifferent to the implications of this "national selfishness" when it also implicated the safety of their own citizens.

Crises have often led to innovation in international cooperation. However, the COVID-19 pandemic was not one such crisis. In this respect at least, the "post-COVID world" resembles the world before—and perhaps will become even worse.

Preparing for the Post-COVID World

Stéphane Dion,
Former Minister of Intergovernmental Affairs,
Environment and Climate Change, and Foreign Affairs

What does our post-COVID-19 world look like? How is humanity recovering from this pandemic and all its economic and social repercussions? These are questions we are all asking. This volume offers answers from some fifty professors. They examine the short- and long-term effects of the pandemic on essential aspects of our future, including not only how to prevent epidemics and better contain them when they do hit but also what has become of democracies grappling with authoritarian and populist pressures; the protection of rights and freedoms and of minorities; the safeguarding of privacy in the face of surveillance technology; the deployment of digital technology and platforms, their regulation, taxation, and effects on public debate; biodiversity protection and the fight against climate change; production chain reliability and the tension between free trade and protectionism; the reduction of wealth inequalities between and within countries; the solvency of states, companies, and individuals; the quest for peace and the avoidance of a new Cold War despite conflict between powers, particularly between the United States and China; multilateralism and how international organizations such as the World Health Organization and the World Trade Organization function; and migratory flows and migrant worker integration.

The authors also remind Canada of its duties. In a world seeking more effective international cooperation, Canada has many strengths, not only with its excellent scientists and researchers—particularly in the field of health—but also more generally as a North American democracy that abuts the powerful United States, is strongly linked to Europe but has also strengthened its ties considerably with Asia; with two official languages with global reach and a multicultural population that gives it a foothold on every continent; with an experienced diplomatic presence at all international forums; with a developed economy that is both technologically advanced and rich in natural resources, including those the world will require to transition successfully to a carbon-neutral economy; with a quarter of the Arctic, the ecological and geostrategic importance of which is growing all the time.

The perspectives the authors develop over the chapters are rich and varied, but if I had to put my finger on a common characteristic, I would say it is the refusal of fatalism. Humanity can bounce back, continue to make progress on many fronts, and remedy the shortcomings the pandemic has brought to light. This is a healthy dose of voluntarism as we grapple with a tragedy that has claimed millions of lives, plunged over a hundred million people into extreme poverty, and locked down populations for months on end.

To preserve our self-confidence, we can examine how humanity has coped with this pandemic in comparison with previous ones. As I write, we are mourning the tragic loss of more than three million people from coronavirus. A century earlier, the pandemic that was erroneously called the "Spanish Flu" claimed somewhere between fifty and one hundred million lives—depending on the estimate—for a world population that was less than two billion at the time. In our world of 7.8 billion people, this would be equivalent to a massacre that could have claimed between 200 and 400 million lives.

The fact is, humanity has made immense progress in terms of medical knowledge, health practices, healthcare systems, and scientific cooperation. We even surprised ourselves by managing to produce vaccines in less than a year.

Let us look beyond the purely medical aspect. From 1970 to 2020, humanity's population doubled, and its wealth increased fivefold. During this period, average global life expectancy rose from fifty-six to seventy-two years. As recently as 1990, almost one in three people did not have access to electricity; this has since been reduced to one in ten. This is undeniable progress that needs to continue.

According to the World Bank, the proportion of people living in extreme poverty (on less than $2 per day) has fallen from one in two (48 percent) in 1970 to less than one in 10 today. This spectacular reduction was unfortunately interrupted by COVID-19, which is estimated to have pushed or kept some 119 to 124 million people in poverty worldwide (Lackner et al. 2021). This humanitarian setback must be corrected as soon as possible through the strong multilateral-backed international solidarity we have gradually built up since 1945 and that we must continue to strengthen in all areas.

Similarly, on the political front, despite geopolitical and economic rivalries between powers, we must find ways to continue making significant progress toward a more peaceful world. While the number of active intrastate conflicts has risen in recent years, mainly due to the actions of violent jihadist groups, the number of victims of these conflicts continues to fall (Pettersson, Högbladh, and Öberg 2019).[1]

Democracies today face many challenges with authoritarian regimes and populist tendencies. But here again, historical perspective gives us courage. According to the International Institute for Democracy and Electoral Assistance, 26 percent of countries were democratic in 1975, compared with 62 percent in 2018. This is impressive progress, in fact the greatest wave of democratization in history, even considering the questionable nature and fragility of many of these democracies. There are now democracies in every region of the world (International Institute for Democracy and Electoral Assistance 2019).

COVID-19 is testing democratic systems around the world. Here again, we may be cautiously optimistic. Admittedly, the fact that the most prominent democratic states are the ones that have declared the highest death rates does not bode well for the prestige of the democratic system. Moreover, it is known that the radical restrictions imposed, on a massive scale, to halt the spread of the pandemic, have resulted in big rollbacks of civil liberties. Rights and freedoms have been curtailed with lockdowns, with the prohibition of public and private gatherings, travel bans, border closures, shop closures, the increasing use of surveillance technologies, large fines, delayed elections, and so forth. All renowned observatories have significantly downgraded 2020 Democracy Index scores from 2019. However, opinion polls have consistently shown strong support for these emergency measures, of course with the understanding that they will be used exclusively for legitimated public health goals and will in no way become permanent.

The economic contraction caused by restrictions imposed to stop the spread of the COVID-19 virus aggravated the instability of fragile democracies. As the health situation deteriorated, hospital infrastructure became overburdened, job losses increased poverty, food prices surge, and tourism—often the backbone of the economy—dried up. The pandemic had a significant impact on women, rolling back many advancements in gender equity. However, these democracies are still alive, and popular protest movements are targeting governments considered incompetent or corrupt, rather than the democratic system itself.

Authoritarian regimes are seizing the opportunity of the pandemic to consolidate their control at the expense of privacy, civil liberties, and rule of law. According to the Economist Intelligence Unit's 2020 Democracy Index, "the biggest regressions occurred in the authoritarian regions.... These regimes took advantage of the global health emergency caused by the coronavirus pandemic to persecute and crack down on dissenters and political opponents" (Economic Intelligence Unit 2020). Similarly, Freedom House found that "settings that already had weak safeguards against abuse of power are suffering the most" (Repucci and Slipowitz 2020).

In Europe, the EU Commission Global Monitor on COVID-19 Impact on Democracy and Human Rights categorized six EU member countries (Bulgaria, Hungary, Poland, Romania, Slovenia, and Slovakia) as experiencing "concerning developments," along with many non-EU European countries.

However, in the well-established democracies, though we certainly saw the rise of disinformation, conspiracy theories, and extremist activism, one may say that overall, the pandemic has not had the effect of radicalizing a large part of the population. There was even a rallying effect around mainstream governments, with—intriguingly—no obvious correlation with the actual effectiveness of these governments in containing the spread of the virus. The approval ratings of incumbent leaders and governments surged at the beginning of the COVID-19 crisis (Bol et al. 2020; Ducke 2020). Of course, what helped to incentivize populations to rally around their ruling leaders are the trillions in cash and liquidity that governments are pumping out, with the hope to ease the pain and safeguard the economy's future. Predictably, over the course of many months and with the effect of weariness, this exceptional support for incumbent governments weakened, but it is far from having disappeared everywhere.

In well-established European democracies, radical parties have been less able to appear as a credible alternative than was the case during the 2008 financial crisis, which lent itself better than the current pandemic to the usual populist blame-game rhetoric against the elites and the experts. The pandemic increased value in an evidence-based and consensus-oriented leadership style, for which most populist demagogues hardly have a profile. As Chancellor Merkel said, the pandemic "is showing the limits of fact-denying populism." The massive efforts in health and social assistance created a unifying effect, while the divisive themes of cultural identity and immigration were put aside by the pandemic emergency.

Of course, there are a lot of unknowns concerning the future. People became inevitably fatigued by the radical socio-administrative restrictions, lockdown, and paralysis of almost all economic activity and impatient with the pace of vaccination. The unlocking of the lockdown was itself fraught with difficulties, while inequality, unemployment, bankruptcies, and debts surged to the forefront of political debate.

Now the pandemic has ceased to be of main concern, the pre-COVID divisive issues are resurfacing: ethno-political tensions will brood and populist politicians will continue to instrumentalize nationalism. The pandemic's economic damage to Latin-American, African, and Middle East countries, coupled with the anticipated economic rebound in North America and Europe, is likely to drive up irregular migration in the coming years. A new migration wave would risk boosting attraction to populist demagogues, to record levels of support.

If there is one issue we must absolutely address, it is that of green recovery. Post-COVID economic recovery must be sustainable and build an economy that is truly more respectful of the planet and the climate. We must not let this opportunity pass us by because we never know when governments will invest so resolutely in the green transition again.

Since 1970, natural resource extraction has tripled, one million of the world's eight million known plant and animal species are threatened with extinction, and ecosystems are deteriorating at an accelerated rate, while climate change is exacerbating this environmental crisis. The world is emitting twice as many greenhouse gases (GHGs) as in 1970 (United Nations Environment Programme 2021). Since 1990, it has emitted more than in the previous 140 years.

According to the International Energy Agency, Global CO_2 emissions declined by 5.8 percent in 2020 because of the economic slowdown caused by the fight against the pandemic but are projected to rebound in 2021, increasing by 6 percent to reach their highest annual level. Global coal demand is expected to increase by 4.5 percent in 2021 and will then exceed 2019 levels (International Energy Agency 2021). If nothing changes, the 2020 drop will have only been a parenthesis in the continued growth of GHG emissions.

We are engaging in self-destructive development, and we need to find the path to sustainable development. From this perspective, the 2015 Paris Agreement was a great diplomatic feat. The problem is that time is running out to stay below the 2°C warming limit scientists recommend we do not exceed. We are already warming at 1°C and are on track for 1.5°C by around 2040 and 3°C by the end of the century, with warming continuing thereafter (Masson et al. 2018)[22]

We need to do more—much more. In December 2020, the Government of Canada released its new climate plan and the Hydrogen Strategy for Canada, and Prime Minister Trudeau announced a tougher Canadian target for 2030 (a 40 percent to 45 percent reduction in emissions from 2005) that will lead our country toward carbon neutrality in 2050. No fewer than 110 countries have pledged to eliminate their emissions by 2050, with China promising to do so by 2060.

Credible action plans are needed to achieve such targets, with carbon pricing the backbone of a good plan. The Government of Canada has courageously proposed to raise the price of carbon pollution from today's C$30 per tonne to C$170 per tonne by 2030. The government's plan was designed to create a powerful incentive for truly sustainable economic prosperity with greater social justice. And social justice—a just transition—is essential to success because nothing will be possible without the support of the people (Dion 2021).

The fight against climate change is also a geostrategic issue. Military and climate experts warn that severe and growing environmental disruptions, aggravated by human-made climate change, are an amplifying factor of conflict and instability (Saghir 2021). To a significant extent, the future of world peace depends on the seriousness with which we will implement assertive post-COVID green recovery plans.

In this final battle against human-induced climate change, we can draw inspiration from the determination with which we fought the coronavirus. However, we need to remember the different nature of these two battles. In the case of the COVID-19 pandemic, governments reacted by placing their populations in a state of transitory irregularity, which is untenable in the long term. We cannot keep people in lockdown forever, deprive hundreds of millions of children of an education, paralyze almost all economic activity, and then ask governments to make up the difference by running up astronomical debts. In the case of the fight against climate change, the aim is to create the opposite of transitory irregularity—a sustainable normality. The aim is to enable a normal life, in which humanity continues to pursue its goals of economic and social progress and justice while maintaining the same opportunities for future generations—therefore, without damaging the natural environment or climate.

In short, if we want to bounce back fully from this pandemic, we need to be cautiously optimistic and devoid of complacency. Determination—free from fatalism—is required. In-depth knowledge of the world and its trends is necessary, which is what makes this book so useful. I hope you enjoy reading it.

Notes

1. This continuing decline in victims of violent conflict tends to confirm the claim that we live in an increasingly peaceful world (for example, see Goldstein 2011 and Pinker 2011).
2. This is an IPCC special report on the impacts of global warming of 1.5°C above pre-industrial levels and related global greenhouse gas emission pathways, in the context of strengthening the global response to the threat of climate change, sustainable development, and efforts to eradicate poverty.

References

Bol, Damien, Marco Giani, André Blais, and Peter John Loewen. 2020. "The Effect of COVID-19 Lockdowns on Political Support: Some Good News for Democracy?" *European Journal of Political Research* 60, no. 2 (May): 497–505. https://doi.org/10.1111/1475-6765.12401.

Dion, Stéphane. 2021. "Practicing Climate Justice: Negotiating Just Transitions in Canada and on the World Stage." In *The Well-Being Transition: Analysis and Policy*, edited by Éloi Laurent, 25–54. London: Palgrave Macmillan.

Ducke, Emile. 2020. "Coronavirus Has Lifted Leaders Everywhere. Don't Expect That to Last." *The New York Times*, April 19, 2020. https://www.nytimes.com/2020/04/15/world/europe/coronavirus-presidents.html.

Economic Intelligence Unit. 2020. *Democracy Index 2020: In Sickness and In Health?* London: Economic Intelligence Unit. https://www.eiu.com/n/campaigns/democracy-index-2020/.

International Energy Agency. 2021. *Global Energy Review: CO2 Emissions in 2021. Global Emissions Rebound Sharply to Highest Ever Level.* Paris: International Energy Agency. https://www.iea.org/reports/global-energy-review-2021?utm_content=buffer5ce8e&utm_medium=social&utm_source=twitter-ieabirol&utm_campaign=buffer.

International Institute for Democracy and Electoral Assistance. 2019. *The Global State of Democracy 2019: Addressing the Ills, Reviving the Promise.* Stockholm: International Institute for Democracy and Electoral Assistance. https://www.idea.int/publications/catalogue/global-state-of-democracy-2019.

Lakner, Christoph, Nishant Yonzan, Daniel Gerszon Mahler, R. Andres Castaneda Aguilar, and Haoyu Wu. 2021. "Updated Estimates of the Impact of COVID-19 on Global Poverty: Looking Back at 2020 and the Outlook for 2021." *World Bank Blogs*, January 11, 2021. https://blogs.worldbank.org/opendata/updated-estimates-impact-covid-19-global-poverty-looking-back-2020-and-outlook-2021.

Masson-Delmotte, Valerie, Panmao Zhai, Hans-Otto Pörtner, Debra C. Roberts, Priyadarshi R. Shukla, Anna Pirani, Wilfran Moufouma-Okia et al., eds. 2018. "Summary for Policymakers." In *Special Report: Global Warming of 1.5°C,* IPCC Special Report. https://www.ipcc.ch/sr15/chapter/spm/.

Pettersson, Therese, Stina Högbladh, and Magnus Öberg. 2019. "Organized Violence, 1989–2018 and Peace Agreements." *Journal of Peace Research* 56, no. 4 (July): 589–603. https://doi.org/10.1177/0022343319856046.

Repucci, Sarah, and Samy Slipowitz. 2020. *Democracy under Lockdown: The Impact of COVID-19 on the Global Struggle for Freedom.* Washington, D.C.: Freedom House. https://freedomhouse.org/sites/default/files/2020-10/COVID-19_Special_Report_Final_.pdf.

Saghir, Jamal. 2021. *Climate Change's Impacts on Conflict: Moving from Acknowledgement to Action.* Potsdam: Potsdam Institute for Climate Impact Research, Berghof Foundation.

United Nations Environment Programme. 2021. *Making Peace with Nature: A Scientific Blueprint to Tackle the Climate, Biodiversity and Pollution Emergencies.* Nairobi: United Nations Environment Programme. https://www.unep.org/resources/making-peace-nature.

Acknowledgements

We thank Amandine Hamon, Lucile Martin, Jana Walkowski and Sylvain Longhais for their help in coordinating and assisting working groups. We also register our appreciation to the Centre de recherche en éthique, the Centre for International Peace and Security Studies, and the Centre d'études et de recherches internationales de l'Université de Montréal for their financial and logistical support.

The Afterworld

Frédéric Mérand and Jennifer Welsh

In the spring of 2020, the world came to a halt. Schools, shops, and restaurants closed. Millions of people lost their jobs. Office staff moved to teleworking while essential workers did double shifts to attend to patients or deliver food. Manufacturing almost stopped. Roads emptied. Airports shut down. This came to be known as the Great Lockdown.

The COVID-19 pandemic is the most significant global crisis since the beginning of the twenty-first century. Its ramifications are sanitary and economic, of course, but also social, technological, environmental, cultural, security-related, psychological, and political. To borrow from the French sociologist Marcel Mauss, we can call it a "total social fact," the likes of which we have not seen since the Second World War: the pandemic encompassed all spheres of human activity and all dimensions of the human experience, from the physiological to the spiritual. And unlike the Second World War, the end of the Cold War, the 2008 Great Recession, or even historically recent disease outbreaks, such as Ebola, not a single country (not China with its so-called "zero-COVID policy," and not even North Korea, the "hermit kingdom") has been able to avoid its consequences.

In some cases, the impact has been swift and dramatic, with the pandemic pushing tens of millions back into poverty and generating extreme food insecurity in communities around the globe. As the Bill & Melinda Gates Foundation put it in their 2020 Goalkeepers Report, when we consider metrics of social and economic development, "we [were] set back about twenty-five years in twenty-five weeks." In other cases, the transformations are still bubbling beneath the surface, and questions swirl as to whether necessary changes in the day-to-day behaviour of populations will be reversed or survive into the post-pandemic period.

Since March 2020, there has been an explosion of analysis on the short-term impact, and possible future consequences, of COVID-19. While downloads of Albert Camus's *The Plague* shot up, parallels were quickly drawn with Stefan Zweig's evocation of Europe's descent into poverty, nationalism, and war during the 1930s in his famous memoir, *The World of Yesterday*. While most commentators were understandably gloomy, some looked for opportunities for positive change. That requires thinking about how, in the "Afterworld," we can work to improve the economy, social justice, the environment, gender relations, health, and political institutions — or, at the very least, to ensure that they do not deteriorate further. Many ideas have been proposed for how to "build back better," in what is probably only the beginning of a global discussion.

In this book, we focus our attention on one level of the challenge: the world itself or, in the language of academia, international relations. Soon after the crisis started, we invited 50 Montréal-based scholars from McGill University and Université de Montréal, but also Université du Québec à Montréal and Concordia University, to meet virtually by Zoom for a marathon of brainstorming sessions. Their mandate was to think together about progressive, pragmatic, and social-science-based ideas that could improve international cooperation, security, and sustainable prosperity after the pandemic is over. We then organized a series of open roundtables where practitioners, decision-makers, activists, and the public were invited to provide their feedback and co-produce knowledge with us. The book you have in your hands is the result of this collective and collaborative undertaking.

The World in 2020

Before we turn to our collaborators' main ideas, and the debates they generated, let us summarize what we know about the (short-term) impact of COVID-19 on international relations.

Revelations

Some global trends were already well in motion before 2020 but were revealed to us with greater clarity by the pandemic. Socio-economic inequalities are a case in point. Between countries, they appear at first glance to have been diminishing since the 1990s, but that is largely a by-product of the rise of the Chinese middle class. Within countries, by contrast, they have been growing in many cases. Overall, as economists such as Thomas Piketty (2019) and Branko Milanović (2016) have shown, the picture is mixed: while millions of people have seen their lives improve in the twenty-first century, especially in the Global South, the top 1 percent of the population has seen its income grow even further—and for many people, either trapped in poverty or part of the stagnant Western middle class, the situation has worsened. Moreover, the nature of socio-economic inequalities has significantly changed. Owning capital generates a larger premium than at any given time since the end of the Second World War. Conversely, unskilled service workers have become comparatively poorer. This was the baseline as we entered the coronavirus crisis, which subsequently underlined the vulnerability of unskilled workers, whether in the formal or the informal sector.

Another global trend highlighted by the pandemic is the growing interdependence of national economies, illustrated by the dense web of global value chains. The shift of manufacturing to China, which took off in the 1990s, had concealed the degree to which the twenty-first-century design, production, and sale of goods and services are integrated globally through intellectual property rights, interoperable logistics, just-in-time communication, regulatory convergence, and financial markets. Extreme specialization means that inputs move around the world constantly: to take an example that is taught in business schools, the components of Apple's iPhone, including intellectual property, come from the United States, Japan, Germany, Taiwan, France, Korea, and, yes, China. In the early days of the pandemic, when countries were faced with shortages of critical medical supplies, there was much talk about onshoring after decades of offshoring. But to date there has been little evidence of a reversal in this secular trend, or the full embrace of "supply chain sovereignty" (Zakaria 2020).

In terms of international politics, the relative decline of the United States had become widely accepted among observers by the beginning of the 2010s. The question that remained was whether the United States would continue to project its soft power vigorously and lead efforts in global cooperation, as the Obama administration had tried to do. But the rise of populism in the "West" and the growing strength of illiberal regimes in the "Rest" put this hope to bed well before 2020. The main victim was the quality of liberal democracy, which according to Freedom House declined every year across countries between 2005 and 2020, because the norms of free elections and the rule of law either weakened in established democracies or were trampled upon in fragile ones (Mounk 2018; Levitsky and Ziblatt 2018). Democratic backsliding was not confined to the few but spread among many and was observed on every continent. While authoritarian regimes like China and Russia became even more authoritarian, countries like Hungary and Turkey, led by democratically elected leaders with autocratic tendencies, came to embody electoral authoritarianism, or "illiberal democracy." As a result, what international relations specialists and diplomats refer to as the "Liberal International Order" was undermined not only by states such as Russia, "but also by voters in the West" (Adler-Nissen and Zarakol 2021). The tumultuous mandate of President Donald Trump (2017–2021) encapsulated these two trends, demonstrating a systematic erosion of U.S. domestic democracy and international legitimacy (Walt 2019).

Finally, COVID-19 reminded us of a simple truth that many had forgotten: the state is a fundamental institution that holds societies together. As Max Weber famously put it, the state owns the monopoly of legitimate violence—but also of citizenship and the protection of populations. Although the state, according to Michael Mann (1984), has the despotic power to impose, it also has the infrastructural power to enable—it has, in the well-known words of Pierre Bourdieu, a "right hand" that constrains and a "left hand" that protects. Governments can shut down factories, close borders, and force people to stay in their homes; but they can also repatriate them from abroad, provide them with free health care, and offer emergency benefits. These exceptional powers were revealed during the crisis, as governments did the unthinkable: curtailing the movement of people or running deficits at 15 percent of the gross domestic product (GDP). Not surprisingly, weaker states coped less well, and many of them exercised more despotic than infrastructural power. The Special Report of the Munich Security Conference in late 2020 went so far as to speak of an "authoritarianism pandemic" running alongside COVID-19, noting a 30 percent increase in government oppression around the world between mid-March and late July (Munich Security Conference 2020, 5).

Catalysis

Then there are the trends that COVID-19 accelerated. This is most obviously the case with the digitalization and virtualization of international relations, where the pandemic has served as a catalyst for further change. The work of corporations, whether small businesses or multinationals, was turned upside down by the home office. Remote working also affected governmental and intergovernmental bureaucracies, which added virtual meetings to the already prevalent use of email communication. As international travel stopped, international meetings, from professional conventions to United Nations (UN) summits, took place online. Like the boardroom and the classroom, the international conference room moved to Zoom. After work, people "went home" to consume unprecedented levels of American culture, most notably on Netflix and Apple, or purchased through Amazon.

The ascent of tech firms largely predated the COVID-19 crisis. They were already gaining in market share and generating eye-popping levels of revenue. But the Great Lockdown gave them a significant boost. As the "real" economy crashed, consumers and investors rushed to the GAFAM (Google, Apple, Facebook, Amazon, Microsoft), while local service economy, tourism, and cultural industries collapsed. In July 2020, the top five tech firms accounted for 22 percent of the S&P 500 stock value (Klebnikov 2021). By locking digital services into people's everyday consumption practices and firms' operations, the pandemic thus accelerated a profound transformation of the capitalist economy, from the sale of products and services to the commodification of data, and to what Shoshana Zuboff (2019) refers to as the rise of "surveillance capitalism." This transformation will benefit workers and firms in the digital economy at the expense of others, who will continue to lose out.

The pandemic thus exposed and amplified many of the underlying dynamics of globalization, particularly in terms of technology (McNamara and Newman 2020). By 2020, it had become clear that the new frontier lay along 5G communications and artificial intelligence. Not surprisingly, innovation within and control of these sectors was also becoming more hotly disputed between China and the United States, constituting a new vector for competition between the world's two great powers and limiting their willingness to cooperate in the face of common challenges. While China cooperated closely with the United States in the wake of the 2008 financial crisis, including within the institutional framework of the G20, it has since developed a huge domestic market and a high-value-added tech sector that is largely autonomous: today, China's largest firms, such as Alibaba or Tencent, rival those based in the United States in size and market value. What is more, China has sought to build its own regional order by signing trade and security deals and extending its control over political developments within its perceived sphere of influence. Beijing's increased confidence has translated into not only a more visible and active presence in international institutions, but also a more "muscular" form of diplomacy designed to further its economic and political interests. The People's Liberation Army has increased in size sevenfold since 1998, bolstering a strategy of nationalist assertiveness that stands in stark contrast with China's previous foreign policy approach—emphasizing quiet bargaining—that prevailed in the early years of the twenty-first century (Chu and Zheng 2020; Bell 2020; Tiberghien 2020).

Two COVID-related factors have heightened and expanded the rivalry between the Chinese and American giants. The first was the politicization of global health. In 2009, China and the United States cooperated during the H1N1 pandemic, by exchanging technology and information about the spread of the disease and accelerating the development of a vaccine. Similarly, in response to the Ebola outbreak in 2014, the two countries—as key UN Security Council members—participated in a collective effort to send aid to West Africa. In 2020, however, the picture was starkly different. While during the earlier SARS outbreak the origin of the disease was viewed as a *scientific* rather than a political issue—with no effort to deny origins or hold particular states accountable—COVID-19 became the focal point for condemnation and competition (Huang 2021). The fact that the coronavirus first erupted in the Chinese region of Wuhan was turned into a rhetorical weapon by Trump in his attempt to shift blame to "Communist China." This framing of the crisis significantly amplified anti-Chinese sentiment, which was already latent in the United States but also in much of the Western world, and tensions between China and the UN undermined the workings of both the World Health Organization (WHO)—which struggled to conduct an independent and transparent investigation of how the pandemic started or to galvanize countries to act together to contain it—as well as the UN Security Council—which could not agree on a resolution to mobilize UN agencies or establish a mechanism to coordinate international response efforts.

Second, performance in responding to COVID-19 became a central feature of the battle over which superpower possessed the best political model. Xi Jinping leveraged his country's record as the first to "tame" the virus in order to embellish his own propaganda about China's rise. China also used the fact that it emerged relatively unscathed from the crisis—managing to achieve 2.3 percent growth in 2020 compared to a 3.5 percent economic contraction in the United States—to champion the superiority of its economic model vis-à-vis the United States' failing policies. This discourse has been echoed in other authoritarian regimes, of course, but also throughout the Global South, where China used "vaccine diplomacy" to assert not only its scientific prowess but also its identity as a responsible great power. In 2021, China assumed an early lead in the race to extend soft power by providing free vaccines to 69 countries across the developing world and commercially exporting to 28 other countries. This was an alternative to the programs of the United States and Europe (Huang 2021). To counteract emerging concerns about the efficacy of Sinovac or the capacity of the Chinese government to fulfill all its "orders," a social media misinformation campaign has been detected which seeks to discredit Western vaccines.

Changing the Game

Finally, we turn to the new trends that COVID-19 initiated. Although trends are, by definition, hard to detect in the space of only a few months, converging pieces of evidence are pointing to important developments in fiscal policy. Since the 1980s, most advanced-economy governments have been focused on fighting inflation at the expense of employment. Since the 1990s, fiscal austerity and the reduction of public spending have been the dominant orthodoxy among professional economists and policymakers (Streeck 2014). This led to a steady decrease in taxes, especially for high-income groups and corporations (Zucman and Saez 2019). After the 2008 financial crisis, many governments engaged in economic stimulus, but they quickly replaced it with fiscal consolidation when the crisis abetted—and sometimes prematurely (Blyth 2013; Tooze 2018).

The 2020 crisis has already proven to be a game changer. In a matter of weeks, the most deeply held convictions about fiscal policy were shattered. Whether "liberal" or "coordinated" market economies, led by conservative or progressive leaders, most Organisation for Economic Co-operation and Development (OECD) governments injected billions of dollars into their economies, generating annual deficits on the order of 5 percent to 15 percent of annual GDP. They expanded unemployment insurance, subsidized jobs and wages, supported businesses, and nationalized firms. In short, they broke every orthodoxy of economic policymaking. Government indebtedness soared. Central banks, for their part, borrowed from the same script they had experimented with after 2012, purchasing bonds and injecting liquidity to keep interest rates to the floor as long as possible with no fear for inflation. Their balance sheet is now higher than at any point in history.

At the time of writing, it is too early to tell whether governments will engage in a new round of fiscal consolidation, decide to live with a much higher level of public debt, or increase taxes. It will likely be a combination of all three options, with different emphases in different countries, depending on capacity and ideology. But the goalposts have been shifted—for at least a little while. There seems to be no optimal debt ceiling; if a large-scale economic stimulus is coordinated, it does not necessarily lead to capital flight. Even in a globalized economy, governments now seem to have the ability to tax and regulate markets much more than the common wisdom had led us to believe.

Exiting the crisis relatively unharmed is not an option that is available to most developing or heavily indebted countries. The pandemic has most likely halted the economic convergence that had been occurring between some of the Global South and the North since the early 2000s. Some countries, notably, China, continue their rise thanks to a large market and well-functioning (albeit authoritarian) institutions. But many others, from Brazil to India, will fall behind again. For the first time since the 1990s, the year 2020 marked an *increase* in global poverty and saw trends related to the pandemic that are exacerbating state fragility in every region of the world. If nothing is done to assist these countries, the goal of sustainable development will look more remote than before.

At the same time, the pandemic challenged previous ways of classifying or judging the success of countries. Some established democracies did much better than others in containing case numbers—think of

South Korea in contrast to the United Kingdom—thus suggesting that "regime type" was a relatively poor predictor for good performance. Similarly, the notion that developed countries have all the answers (a trope that was already declining in credibility before COVID-19) was palpably hard to sustain. When it came to fighting the virus, developed Western states proved that they had much to learn from some developing states, thereby suggesting that, going forward, the relationship between developed and developing countries cannot be a "one way street" (Munich Security Conference 2020, 3).

Finally, COVID-19—unlike other pandemics of the post-Cold War period—has been overwhelmingly viewed through a security lens. Despite all the talk of the need for cooperation, and of pandemic preparedness and response as a global public good, all countries have depicted the virus as a form of existential threat requiring exceptional measures. In the United States, then-President Trump invoked the Defense Production Act to mobilize the COVID-19 response and appointed a four-star general as the director of "Operation Warp Speed" (the plan for vaccine development and roll-out). Even in Canada, a retired general, Rick Hillier, was tasked with getting Ontario ready for vaccine distribution. But as Yanzhong Huang argues, this tendency of states to place themselves on a "war-footing" appears to have relieved them of their *moral* duties towards others and to have motivated their descent into a competitive scramble for critical medical supplies and active pharmaceutical ingredients (Huang 2021). The most obvious manifestation of this trend has been so-called vaccine nationalism, whereby wealthy countries strike separate deals with major producers to secure priority access, seemingly oblivious to the reality that the virus will only be conquered when the global population gains immunity.

Status Quo

Among all these revelations, accelerations, and initiations, there are a great many things that COVID-19 did *not* change in international relations. In terms of geopolitics, the competitive dynamic between the United States and China, with Russia and Europe playing minor roles, was not fundamentally affected by the pandemic. While the soft power of both these dominant nations was initially dented in significant ways by their respective responses to the spread of the virus (Rudd 2020), the overall balance of power between them was not altered. As Daniel Drezner (2020) argues, this suggests that the pandemic will likely not be viewed as a key "inflection point" in their relationship. By and large, the delicate strategic situation also persists in Central Asia, sub-Saharan Africa, the Arctic, and the South China Sea. The nuclear order was already unravelling before the crisis, as the United States and Russia pulled out of arms limitation deals that China did not even want to join, and the possibility for escalation from conventional to nuclear confrontation between other nuclear-armed states—most notably India and Pakistan—remains worryingly real.

In terms of broader global issues, while the coronavirus may have temporarily replaced climate change as the number one "wicked problem," the environment is expected to continue as the main policy challenge of our generation. Similarly, violent conflict—whether perpetuated by government forces, rebel groups and insurgents, terrorist organizations, or criminal networks—continues to imperil civilians and reverse economic and social development. It is true that some non-state armed groups have exploited the pandemic to extend their reach over territories and populations, but the deeper causes of conflict are stubbornly consistent. Turning to migration, its main drivers have also continued, as witnessed by the continued flow of populations to the southern U.S. border. While the movement of peoples may have slowed its pace, this deceleration is not expected to last once borders are reopened. Lastly, despite the emergence of potent anti-mask and anti-vaccine movements, populist forces do not seem to have either intensified or lost steam as a result of the pandemic (Bickerton and Accetti 2021). Having substituted scientific experts for immigrants as their main object of distrust, they remain a profound challenge to the ongoing legitimacy of governments around the world. The list of important dimensions of human activity that did not change as a result of COVID-19 is endless.

Dilemmas for the Near Future

Of course, most of us hope for a fairer, safer, cleaner, and more prosperous future. We wish that decision-makers around the world would view solidarity with others as being not only part of their duty, but also an integral aspect of their self-interest. In this book, our colleagues have put forward a number of tangible ways to get closer to attaining that hope, often despite, but sometimes thanks to, the COVID-19 crisis. In general, they call for more international cooperation rather than less, a greater concern for the vulnerable and the disenfranchised, the audacity to rethink political, economic, and social structures of inequality, the creation of new rights and resources, and innovative solutions to tackle new challenges — for example, harnessing technology or tax competition for social benefit rather than letting seemingly indomitable forces run the show.

Yet, there are two obstacles that could potentially put the brakes on the realization of these proposals. The first is the power of certainty and tradition. While moments of crisis can bring change — both nationally and internationally — history tells us that not all such moments are seized. Those who wish for, or benefit from, the perpetuation of the status quo are plentiful. Whether genuine political, economic, and social transformation emerges from the chaos of crisis depends on a host of factors, including, of course, bold and principled leadership.

The second is the reality that not all good ideas work in tandem. There is no denying that there will be trade-offs, and that many strong proposals may either come into conflict with each other or face real constraints. Let us take the environment and the global economy. The Great Lockdown has shown that economic collapse is exactly what the planet might need: less production, less consumption, less commuting, and less international travel have all temporarily reduced our carbon footprint. Some observers have concluded from that experience that "deglobalization," or a slowing down of globalization, may be good for the environment. But to fund healthcare systems and economic support programs, to combat unemployment, and later to bring down public debt, governments will be more tempted than ever to stimulate economic activity at all costs. How do we strike the balance?

Another dilemma concerns the development and deployment of technology. It is quite likely that humans will continue to substitute some face-to-face interactions with digital interfaces. During the pandemic, people spent more time than ever on their screens. Doing so enabled them to continue to work, attend school, entertain themselves, and connect with family and friends. Technology has also allowed scientists to cooperate on the global search for a vaccine in real time; while populations in some developed countries lament the pace of vaccination, there is no denying the remarkable feat of ingenuity and cooperation that saw the world start the delivery of new vaccines within nine months of the appearance of COVID-19. Information technology and the harnessing of big data have also allowed governments and private firms to roll out technological solutions to trace the

virus or track mobility. But these welcome developments have understandably faced a barrage of criticisms from human rights activists
and those concerned with privacy. The controversies that erupted
during the pandemic herald some of the pressing questions that societies will need to collectively address in the coming years as technologies become ever more sophisticated.

We noted above that the crisis reminded many of us of the
enduring centrality of the state in the functioning of human societies. During the worst episodes of the pandemic, governments made
all the critical decisions to halt the spread of the virus, such as when
and how to "lock down," and delivered critical health and economic
supports for those in need. In most jurisdictions, the "public health
advisor" emerged from relative obscurity to become a prominent and
trusted public figure. But for a long-term solution, all eyes were on
vaccine research—and that was conducted by private firms, for private gain. In the developing world, where governments often did not
have the resources to purchase vaccine shots, let alone regulate big
pharma, private philanthropic foundations—working with a handful
of governments—stepped in to pick up the slack. This experience begs
the question of how to organize and oversee public-private partnerships when it comes to addressing basic human needs.

There is a final, delicate dilemma raised by the contributions in
this book. During the pandemic, holding the citizenship of a specific
country became the most valued commodity of all. Based on their citizenship, expatriates could be repatriated but guest workers could be
expelled; people could receive precious social benefits or be denied
them; they could happen to live in countries that had (more or less)
the situation under control, or be left to their own devices. As governments try to cushion the social impact of the Great Lockdown and
rebuild their economies, the benefits of a passport—or in some cases,
the "right" passport—will remain profound. Being a refugee or a
migrant, especially coming from the Global South, was already difficult before March 2020. It has only become worse. While it may be
tempting to advocate for open borders, there is currently no alternative to the nation-state as the provider of the cherished good of economic and personal security. But this means that millions of human
beings will be more trapped than ever before in the confines of territories where they do not wish to stay, because they are poor or persecuted, or simply because they want to marry someone of a different
nationality.

Proposals for Change

So what are the progressive, pragmatic, and social-science-based ideas that our colleagues put forward to improve international cooperation, security, and sustainable prosperity? There are too many to be listed here, therefore, while we invite you to read individual chapters, allow us to summarize the three main "packages" of ideas.

The first package revolves around *democratization*. This includes the democratization of international organizations, which should go hand in hand with greater supranational authority when there is collective agreement on what should be done. Many analysts argue that the WHO had all the authority it needed to declare a "Public Health Emergency of International Concern" early on in the crisis and to collect disease-event information that might have contained the virus, but that it showed excessive deference to state sovereignty. But to these weaknesses we must add deficiencies in how such bodies develop recommendations and are held accountable to their key stakeholders. The pandemic has shown more broadly that several international organizations suffer from a lack of "input legitimacy" (Scharpf 1998) vis-à-vis nation states, which significantly hampers their ability to perform. More and more, democratization entails the imperative of inclusion. This means including beneficiaries, for example of health or migration policy, as well as ethnic, gender, and sexual minorities and other vulnerable groups. But empowerment also concerns states and communities that have been marginalized from global governance so far. Consequently, part of the challenge of our time is to address global public contestation (Börzel and Zürn 2021). While our discussion focused on the global level, many groups emphasize the importance of grassroots solutions based on field or community experience. This is particularly true for the delivery of health services. The "localization" imperative thus entails a willingness to engage more deeply with civil society organizations and even, in some cases, with local armed groups who have been on the front lines of delivering vital services to populations.

The second package of ideas insists on the significance of *creating, strengthening, or reaffirming human rights,* such as the rights of health workers and migrants. This may require, in the case of information technology, overhauling our justice system to respond to the new challenges of our digital lives and the normalization of a state of emergency, as crisis management becomes a new form of government.

Relatedly, our colleagues propose new policy instruments, for instance, to tax pollution and digital firms, to monitor human rights gaps, to increase economic policy coordination, or to share the lessons of intergovernmental governance across countries. Some of these could help support new resources to mitigate economic hardship (in the short term) and redress inequities (in the long term) vis-à-vis the developing world.

A final set of ideas simply counsels balance and perspective: let us not focus all our attention on the pandemic. Security and development are challenges in their own right, and diverting resources away from these pressing problems, in order to fight the virus, will end up undermining whatever global progress has been made since the end of the Cold War. Similarly, for many countries around the world, COVID-19 is not viewed as the most urgent health issue or crisis, and the diversion of resources to this disease comes at the expense of continued progress on other health threats to their populations. In short, both internationally and domestically, there have been huge *opportunity costs* incurred while mounting a response to COVID-19. The most significant among them have been borne by the world's children: millions of them have experienced school closures at critical periods in their development, with effects that will be felt for many years to come. At the same time, their parents—predominantly mothers—who cared for them and tried to fill education gaps have seen their own careers and well-being suffer.

Canada and COVID-19

We conclude with some reflections on how our own country, Canada, managed the trends we have outlined, and what Canadian citizenship has meant during this pandemic. In the "reveal" category, Canadians have been reminded of the pros and cons of our federal system, where provincial responsibility for health means greater sensitivity to regional needs and variation, but where centralized direction and common standards often prove elusive just when they were needed most. We have also witnessed the degree to which relatively high levels of trust in government in this country translate into strong levels of compliance with the directives of public health authorities.

But the pandemic has also revealed the costs of earlier political decisions. These choices largely eliminated homegrown vaccine production and severely weakened our previously world-class pandemic surveillance and response capacity. To these uncomfortable truths, we must add the growing questions about Canada's reputation for generosity and cooperation. Critics have noted the fact that far more vaccines were pre-ordered for the Canadian population than were actually needed—ten doses per citizen—thereby making it harder for developing countries to access their required doses in a timely manner. In addition, while Canada was a generous financial backer of the COVAX initiative to create an equitable system for distributing vaccines around the world, Canada was also criticized for its early decision, unique among G7 countries, to procure 1.9 million doses from this facility. While technically within the letter of the COVAX agreement (which included the option of a "self-financed" portion of vaccines for wealthier countries), it was difficult to meet the charge that Canada was prioritizing its lower-risk populations ahead of higher-risk populations in poorer countries. As our contributors to this volume all suggest, a Canadian passport, with all the citizenship privileges that it entails, will continue to be a valuable commodity in the global context of inequality and instability that will mark the "Afterworld."

References

Adler-Nissen, Rebecca, and Ayse Zarakol. 2021. "Struggles for Recognition: The Liberal International Order and the Merger of Its Discontents." *International Organization* 75, no. 2 (Spring): 611–634. https://www.cambridge.org/core/journals/international-organization/article/struggles-for-recognition-the-liberal-international-order-and-the-merger-of-its-discontents/2CA314390EAC48EA619D7834C3A71CA4.

Bell, Daniel. 2020. "Towards an Asian Regional Order Led by China and India." In *The Decline of the Western-Centric World and the Emerging New Global Order*, edited by Yu-Han Chu and Yongnian Zheng, 326–354. London: Routledge.

Bickerton, Christopher, and Carlo Invernizzi Accetti. 2021. *Technopopulism. The New Logic of Democratic Politics.* Oxford: Oxford University Press.

Bill & Melinda Gates Foundation. 2020. "COVID-19. A Global Perspective." *2020 Goalkeepers Report.* September 2020. https://www.gatesfoundation.org/goalkeepers/report/2020-report/#GlobalPerspective.

Börzel, Tanja, and Michael Zürn. 2021. "Contestations of the Liberal International Order: From Liberal Multilateralism to Postnational Liberalism." *International Organization* 75, no. 2 (Spring): 282–305. https://www.cambridge.org/core/journals/international-organization/article/

contestations-of-the-liberal-international-order-from-liberal-multilater-alism-to-postnational-liberalism/7CE3FD0F629D18BE45EB9C7AC7095 4AA.

Blyth, Mark. 2013. *Austerity: The History of a Dangerous Idea.* Oxford: Oxford University Press.

Chu, Yu-Han, and Yongnian Zheng, ed. 2020. *The Decline of the Western-Centric World and the Emerging New Global Order.* London: Routledge.

Drezner, Daniel. 2020. "The Song Remains the Same: International Relations After COVID-19." *International Organization* 74, no. S1 (December): E18–E35. https://www.cambridge.org/core/journals/international-organization/article/song-remains-the-same-international-relations-after-covid19/C0FAED193AEBF0B09C5ECA551D174525.

Huang, Yanzhong. 2021. "Why the World Lost to the Pandemic." *Foreign Affairs,* January 28, 2021. https://www.foreignaffairs.com/articles/united-states/2021-01-28/why-world-lost-pandemic.

Klebnikov, Sergeï. 2021. "Apple, Microsoft, Amazon, Google and Facebook Make Up a Record Chunk of the S&P 500. Here's Why That Might Be Dangerous." *Forbes*, July 24, 2021. https://www.forbes.com/sites/sergeiklebnikov/2020/07/24/apple-microsoft-amazon-google-and-facebook-make-up-a-record-chunk-of-the-sp-500-heres-why-that-might-be-dangerous/?sh=18c162c44f6b.

Levitsky, Steven, and Daniel Ziblatt. 2018. *How Democracies Die.* New York: Crown.

Mann, Michael. 1984. "The Autonomous Power of the State: Its Origins, Mechanisms, and Results." *Archives européennes de sociologie* 25 (2): 185–213.

McNamara, Kathleen R., and Abraham L. Newman. 2020. "The Big Reveal: COVID-19 and Globalization's Great Transformations." *International Organization* 74, no. S1 (December): E59–E77. https://www.cambridge.org/core/journals/international-organization/article/big-reveal-covid19-and-globalizations-great-transformations/56E7E235EE971A9E393CDFA4484CE561.

Milanović, Branko. 2016. *Global Inequality: A New Approach for the Age of Globalization.* Cambridge: Harvard University Press.

Mounk, Yascha. 2018. *The People vs. Democracy: Why Our Freedom Is in Danger and How to Save It.* Cambridge: Harvard University Press.

Munich Security Conference. 2020. "Polypandemic." Special Edition of the Munich Security Report on Development, Fragility, and Conflict in the Era of Covid-19. https://securityconference.org/en/publications/msr-special-editions/stability-2020/.

Piketty, Thomas. 2019. *Capital et idéologie.* Paris: Le Seuil.

Rudd, Kevin. 2020. "The Coming Post-COVID Anarchy: The Pandemic Bodes Ill for Both American and Chinese Power—and for the Global Order."

Foreign Affairs, May 6, 2020. https://www.foreignaffairs.com/articles/united-states/2020-05-06/coming-post-covid-anarchy.

Scharpf, Fritz. 1998. "Interdependence and Democratic Legitimation." MPIfG Working Paper No. 98/2. http://www.mpifg.de/pu/workpap/wp98-2/wp98-2.html.

Streeck, Wolfgang. 2008. *Buying Time. The Delayed Crisis of Democratic Capitalism.* London: Verso.

Tiberghien, Yves. 2020. "Asia's Rise and the Transition to a Post-Western Global Order." In *The Decline of the Western-Centric World and the Emerging New Global Order,* edited by Yu-Han Chu and Yongnian Zheng, 357–378. London: Routledge.

Tooze, Adam. 2019. *Crashed: How a Decade of Financial Crises Changed the World.* London: Penguin.

Walt, Stephen. 2019. "The End of Hubris and the New Age of American Restraint." *Foreign Affairs,* April 16, 2019. https://www.foreignaffairs.com/united-states/end-hubris.

Zakaria, Fareed. 2020. *Ten Lessons for a Post-Pandemic World.* New York: Penguin.

Zuboff, Shoshana. 2019. *The Age of Surveillance Capitalism.* New York: Public Affairs.

Zucman, Gabriel, and Emmanuel Saez. 2019. *The Triumph of Injustice. How the Rich Dodge Taxes and How to Make Them Pay.* New York: W.W. Norton.

CHAPTER 1

Global Governance in the Wake of COVID-19

Jennifer Welsh, Frédéric Mérand, T.V. Paul,
Vincent Pouliot, and Jean-Philippe Thérien

Let's engage in a thought experiment. What if, in mid-January 2020, a global cooperative mechanism to contain and mitigate the spread of COVID-19 had been available? What if, following a determination by the World Health Organization (WHO) that there was a risk of a pandemic *and* a directive from that organization for all governments to activate procedures for a coordinated response, the International Civil Aviation Organization (ICAO) had grounded all aircraft and restricted international travel? Even if one might quibble with the precise details of this scenario, it is certainly one that is within the realm of human possibility.

Yet, once we start to reflect on why this did not occur, we also understand the complexities and inherent challenges of global governance. To begin, we would quickly observe that the body that regulates civil aviation—ICAO, based in Montréal—does not have the authority to shut down international air travel. Second, we would realize that there is no joint crisis mechanism between such a body and the Geneva-based WHO. Moreover, we would acknowledge that WHO's power to direct sovereign states to act on the International Health Regulations (IHR)—designed to serve as both an early warning tool and a mechanism for coordinating responses to pandemics—is heavily constrained (Louis 2020).

Indeed, the limits of global governance reflect a wider reluctance on the part of sovereign states to transfer substantial authority to international organizations. While the director-general of WHO has the power to declare a "public health emergency of international concern" (or PHEIC), thereby activating states' obligations on surveillance, cooperation, and information sharing, states also retain the right to either apply national health measures going beyond WHO's recommendations, or to breach some of their obligations when they consider it "necessary." In addition, WHO, along with a number of other agencies and inter-governmental bodies linked to the United Nations (UN) system, struggles to galvanize political support and resources for *preventive* action—the effectiveness of which seems to be perennially challenging to "prove." Most of the action in global governance remains focused on either crisis response or, at best, escalation prevention, rather than on strategic actions to develop collective resilience.

And finally, when we extend our consideration of "what if" even further, we find that our current global governance architecture, including organizations like ICAO and WHO, are frequently politicized and instrumentalized by governments that benefit from the lack of public scrutiny and accountability beyond the nation-state. Even if scientists and international officials had reached a clear consensus on measures such as the shutdown of air travel—and this is a big "if," given that science rarely leads us to definitive or homogenous public policy guidance—there would undoubtedly have been diplomatic pressures counteracting the push for such measures. For example, air travel companies and corporations would have pushed back against any early effort that is detrimental to their activities.

The fascinating, but also tragic, reality of global governance is that we can frequently imagine a technical solution to a problem we have clearly identified, and yet can easily see why that solution (to carry the theme of air travel further) "won't fly." If COVID-19 teaches us, or reminds us, of anything, it is that global governance challenges cannot be solved by purely technocratic answers. Of course, science and expertise have an important role to play, but governance decisions necessarily rely on different values and entail unequal and unintended consequences. If we are right, we thus need to pay attention to the politics of global governance.

COVID-19 as Amplifier of Tensions in Global Governance

Once the coronavirus morphed from the dangerous outbreak of a communicable disease into a pandemic, it was clear that it called for coordination, at the very least, to facilitate an adequate supply of healthcare and testing equipment, to share test treatment results and the development of vaccines, to ensure transparent and dynamic information on the evolution of the virus, and to amplify and synchronize fiscal action to address the economic impacts of the crisis. Nevertheless, on 25 March 2020, when the leaders of G7 countries met by video conference to discuss the COVID-19 pandemic and its unfolding effects, the meeting merely served as a forum for showcasing deep divisions within the international community, rather than as an impetus for global policy cooperation. Not only was there no final communiqué from the gathering, but leaders reportedly could not even agree on what to call the epidemic. In a context of rising U.S.-China tensions, Trump administration officials insisted on calling it the "Wuhan virus," putting the blame on the Chinese region where COVID-19 was first identified. Although the disposition to meaningfully cooperate was generally in short supply, it is worth asking whether, under a different U.S. president, the G7 would have mounted a more timely and effective response—if only to underscore that many global institutions are vulnerable to the spoiling effects of the "bad apple" problem.

The G20—which represents 80 percent of global economic output and two thirds of the world's population, and which was a lead actor in confronting the 2008 financial crisis—fared only marginally better. At the end of March, G20 leaders pledged their commitment to coordinate public health and financial measures and to support the work of WHO.

In particular they promised to inject, collectively, $5 trillion into the global economy to cushion the impact of COVID-19.[1] Overwhelmingly, however, national action—including a mobilization of financial resources that was widely asymmetric depending on state capacities—dwarfed efforts in international cooperation. In fact, despite the pledge to facilitate trade, many G20 governments did not explicitly call for an end to export bans that many countries—including France, Germany, and India—placed on drugs and medical supplies. Subsequent examples of self-interested behaviour included early efforts by the United States to hoard medicines and, in recent months, the emergence of "vaccine nationalism." At the end of January 2021, a year after the pandemic had begun, none of the approximately 68 million doses of vaccines that had been administered had been provided in low-to-middle income countries, leading the Director-General of

WHO, Tedros Adhanom Ghebreyesus, to claim that the world was "on the brink of catastrophic moral failure" (Huang 2021).

Beyond pointing to the limitations in intergovernmental cooperation, however, it is also crucial to understand the ways in which the evolution of global governance has, in part, created the breeding ground for a pandemic like COVID-19. In recent decades, steps taken in the name of governance innovation have had unintended consequences. By harnessing the contribution of private donors to provide global public goods, multi-stakeholder partnerships (MSPs) aim to be more inclusive, but they inadvertently undermine the strength of broader national capacities. The Global Alliance for Vaccines and Immunization (GAVI), for instance, redirects precious resources away from the public health infrastructure in the Global South, and channels them instead towards segmented programs that follow external actors' preferences. The World Bank and other lending institutions have also had a role to play (whether consciously or inadvertently) in weakening public healthcare systems, which are the core basis for responding to pandemics. These trends in privatization raise the question of who bears responsibility for the shape of contemporary global governance, and who should be accountable for its renovation.

Finally, the unfolding of the COVID-19 pandemic unsettled our understanding of what it is to be a "good citizen" of global governance. Sweden is the illustrative case: though by many measures it is one of the most admired countries in the world, it resisted most of the policies of confinement that other nations implemented. What may have been the right or the wrong decision should serve as a reminder that sovereignty is not just a stumbling block on the way to the greater "good" of international cooperation. It also serves as a protective principle for the self-determination of different political communities. It thus fosters diversity of experiences as well as mutual learning and productive emulation, that which organizations such as WHO function as a conduit. Given the outcome of our thought experiment— which emphasized the realities of uncertainty and the need for politics and deliberation—a "one-size-fits-all" policy response throughout the world would probably have been undesirable. Rather than hand-wringing about sovereignty's deleterious effects, we should thus remember that it can and should be functional in helping contemporary societies to work towards effective solutions to global challenges.

Unfit for Purpose?

In addition to the widespread health crisis, the pandemic had a devastating economic impact, pushing the world into its worst economic crisis since the Great Depression, throwing millions of people into food insecurity and making 2020 the first year since the 1990s in which global poverty, pre-social transfers, *increased* (World Bank 2020, 5; Munich Security Conference 2021, 12). The pandemic also heightened the crisis of living standards in the developing world, where the economic effects of the pandemic were felt most acutely. For example, remittances, which comprise approximately 20 percent of the gross domestic product (GDP) for developing countries as a whole, were projected to drop by US$109 billion in 2020 (United Nations 2020). The social, fiscal, economic, and political impacts of COVID-19 could take development back by a decade or more, wiping out gains on several of the economic Sustainable Development Goals (SDGs) and making other SDGs—such as those related to health, sanitation, and global cooperation—more difficult to achieve. At the same time, if pandemic-era trends of economic isolationism continue, the seeming global tide of protectionism will grow in strength, placing further stress on the multilateral trading system. As of October 2020, for example, nine jurisdictions around the world had imposed export controls on medical supplies (Munich Security Conference 2020).

As a result of these interlocking crises—what the Munich Security Conference has referred to as a "polypandemic"—we have been bombarded with the refrain that COVID-19 represented a "game changer" for the ways in which societies function and interact. The influential American writer Robert Kaplan (2020), for example, suggested that the pandemic will stand as the "historical marker between the first phase of globalization and the second," while economist and former U.S. Treasury official Lawrence Summers (2020) goes further and argues that the dramatic events it initiated will be a "hinge in history." Yet, what is striking from the particular perspective of international relations is the degree to which the pandemic represents not radical change, but rather an amplifier of pre-existing deep tensions and pathologies. As the veteran U.S. foreign policy analyst Richard Haass (2020) put it, COVID-19 appears to be less of a turning point and more a "way station along the road that the world has been traveling" over the past two decades. For French academic Jean-Baptiste Jeangène Vilmer (2020), the pandemic "confirms and exacerbates pre-existing trends" towards less freedom, less openness, and less prosperity. "There will be no world after," he concludes.

In short, in the domain of global governance, the pandemic has acted more as a "big reveal" (McNamara and Newman 2020). The governance malaise it highlighted includes institutions held hostage to geopolitical rivalry, particularly between the United States and China; a failure to coordinate policies in timely and effective ways, for example on humanitarian relief in contexts of conflict; an inability to find common solutions to distribute critical goods and resources or to share burdens, for example on climate change; and a lack of accountability for failure to abide by rules and standards, for example for the digital age. Moreover, COVID-19 emerged in a context where globalization had profoundly shaped social identities and the functioning of political authority. In fact, Romain Lecler (2020) argued early on in the spread of the virus, the pandemic is itself a product of globalization.

We define global governance as "the totality of institutions, policies, norms, procedures and initiatives through which States and their citizens try to bring more predictability, stability and order to their responses to transnational challenges" (United Nations 2014, vi). Created mainly through intergovernmental collaboration, global governance is also increasingly driven by non-state actors (including international bureaucracies such as the UN Secretariat, non-governmental organizations such as Médecins Sans Frontières, private companies and organizations such as the Gates Foundation, and multi-stakeholder groups such as the Internet Corporation for Assigned Names and Numbers). Thanks to global governance, letters and packages can be posted worldwide (the Universal Postal Union is one of the oldest international organizations), cash-strapped governments can be given last-resort loans to pay their nurses, teachers, and doctors, and peace operations can be deployed to prevent civilian casualties in conflict-ridden regions. But the limitations and flaws of global governance also stand in shocking contrast with the size of today's global challenges.

Some have rightly noted that the traditional architecture of international cooperation created in the wake of the Second World War has been struggling for some time to meet these contemporary challenges. The stalled Doha trade round, the limited gains of the most recent rounds of climate negotiations, the mounting stress upon the nuclear non-proliferation treaty, or the limited success in reforming the governance of refugees and migration, all seem to suggest that multilateralism was already "on life support."[2] The inability to collectively coordinate responses to the coronavirus, and the economic and social crisis it prompted, is only one further manifestation of the tendency to fall back on national solutions rather than effective collaboration.

One of the most vivid examples is the UN Security Council. During the 2014 Ebola crisis, the Council passed a landmark decision (Resolution 2177),[3] which both called for and galvanized a number of collective actions—including the repurposing of a UN peace operation in West Africa. This stands in stark contrast to its response to what Secretary-General António Guterres told its Member States in April 2020 was "the gravest test" to the UN since "the founding of this organization." Over the past decade, and in particular in relation to the crisis in Syria, growing geopolitical divisions have severely undermined the Council's capacity to discharge its responsibility to manage international threats to peace and security and take timely and decisive action. During March 2020, when China held the rotating presidency of the Council, it did not even place the virus on the agenda for discussion. Meanwhile, the United States focused its diplomacy on a futile effort to have the Council pass a resolution effectively blaming China for the outbreak of the pandemic.

This last illustration points to a key feature of the structure of world power that makes effective global governance more difficult to achieve now than at any time since 1990: the rise of China and relative decline of the United States. Sino-U.S. rivalry, which has grown considerably since Xi Jinping became secretary-general of the Communist Party in 2012 and was exacerbated by the Trump administration's overtly competitive China policy, is infecting virtually every domain of international relations, from trade and finance, to development assistance, to technology and digital platforms. Moving away from the "peaceful rise" strategy of previous decades, China is increasingly assertive on the world stage. This includes greater contributions to UN missions, but also more frequent use of its veto power in the Security Council and a more concerted campaign to impose its will on UN bodies. Greater assertiveness has also been manifest in China's "wolf warrior diplomacy," in which it threatens or retaliates against countries that criticize its policies. Trump's United States, for its part, deliberately antagonized China—for example, through tariffs and sanctions—and fuelled latent anti-Chinese sentiment in the United States. As a result of this competitive dynamic, and compounded by Russia's geopolitical tactics, global governance had turned into a form of siege warfare even before the pandemic. Social media simply offered the contending parties one more powerful tool to vilify or interfere in one another's affairs.

Five Weaknesses in Contemporary Multilateralism

A common critique of multilateralism that prevailed prior to COVID-19 is that the design of the key post-1945 institutional architecture fails to reflect the growing power and influence of non-Western states. This first weakness is particularly problematic for the legitimacy of multilateral institutions, as the "special responsibilities" assigned to great powers after the Second World War are increasingly questioned by those who believe the current hierarchies built into many international organizations can no longer be defended—either on empirical or normative grounds (Archarya 2018). Yet, at the same time, the established powers' interests and priorities have arguably become even more entrenched in the system and seem unlikely to budge. As a result, those states that feel marginalized within that system insist, first, that this order reflects historical power disparities and, second, that not all equally benefitted from the system of organizations, rules, and relationships that regulated political, security, and economic cooperation for the last 75 years.

The second weakness of contemporary multilateralism—its reliance on particular representations of power and interests—means that it maintains a system whereby a consensus among sovereign governments is required to advance collective policy on global problems, even when that consensus effectively results in the lowest common denominator. It also under-represents additional, non-state actors that are critical players in many stages of the policy-making cycle—whether we consider cities, groups of transnational experts, civil society organizations, or, in some cases, private businesses—thereby underplaying their possible contribution but also avoiding their accountability for underperformance.

The current malaise in global governance, however, extends even deeper. The normative divisions that pervade the global stage go a long way in accounting for the difficulty in achieving collective action. During the 1990s and 2000s, when the world was being reconfigured after the Cold War, it may have appeared as though a liberal, rules-based international order was the only game in town. But as China's growing leadership among African and Asian nations suggests, not everyone on the world stage aspires to the same thing. Moreover, it is important to note that values at the global level are not simply plural or diverse. Just as in domestic politics, they are also inherently conflictual, often leading to intense debates and political clashes. Building on these insights, we argue that the definition of global problems, the establishment of collective goals, and the evaluation of joint remedies generate conflict because all these processes involve making choices — not only among possible actions to be taken, but also between distinct values. As such, global governance solutions are almost always the product of competing normative systems.

The fourth element of the current crisis within the multilateral system is the retreat of one of its key architects, the United States, and its reluctance to work within a rules-based and cooperative framework. This threatens to create a situation in which some of the most critical players simply exit rather than voice their disapproval. Here, it is important to note that the current suspicion of internationalism within the ruling political elite in the United States, which runs counter to many of the ideas that inspired the creation of institutions in the wake of the Second World War, does not lie solely at the feet of the Trump administration and has survived, even if in a different form, under the Biden administration.

A final challenge for contemporary global governance, which well predates COVID-19, is the draining of legitimacy from international institutions. In large part, this is a result of the perception — on both the right and the left — that global politics is enacted by and for the elite, which benefits from economic globalization. The profound levels of inequality both between and within societies, which were exacerbated by the 2008 financial crisis, have contributed to a discourse against the practices and values of international cooperation, and generated calls to address the imbalance between the "winners" and "losers" of globalization as well as to devote greater attention to domestic prosperity and security. As a result, global structures today attract easy scapegoating from a variety of actors and have become victims of domestic political dynamics in a number of countries — which only further de-legitimizes them.

The Challenges and Opportunities of COVID-19

The Nobel prize-winner Paul Romer once quipped that a "crisis is a terrible thing to waste."[4] And indeed, experience does show us that crises can sometimes lead to productive policy change and governance innovation. This was true in terms of the domestic, regional, and international transformations of the early post-1945 period, as well as, to a lesser extent, in the nuclear realm in the 1970s. But in other cases, reform and innovation have not followed episodes of crisis. In fact, while crises are relatively numerous in the *longue durée* of history, meaningful transformations of economic, social, and political orders are much less common. This is so for two reasons.

First, as Sheri Berman (2020) has reminded us, it is much easier to generate discontent against an old system than to build a clear consensus on a new way forward. This is why revolutionary moments, like that of 1848, do not always fulfill their potential. The "key determinants of whether crises and discontent trigger transformation," she writes, "are [ultimately] political." Without a clear purpose and concrete plans, opposition groups with alternative visions fall into infighting—as happened within the European left in the 1920s and 1930s—and without political power behind good ideas to ensure their implementation, "the status quo can stumble on."

A second and related explanation, drawn from the work of Ronald Krebs (2015), is that crisis periods activate, and over time can amplify, the psychological need for certainty. Even though multiple narratives about new policies and approaches circulate, previously hegemonic ideas and paradigms can persist—despite the evidence seeming to suggest they are no longer fit for their original purpose—as people seek out stability and "closure." If rhetorically powerful actors are able to argue for a recognizable and predictable order, with only minor tinkering, the opportunity for transformation may pass, and policy options that lack strong "narrative grounding" are ignored or quickly rejected (Krebs 2015, 44).

So, will retrenchment or innovation win out in this crisis? Given our earlier discussion of the weaknesses of multilateralism, it is easy to leap to the conclusion that the pandemic will only make things worse. The experience of confronting COVID-19, both within countries and in global policy-making forums, has given an even bigger platform to "short-termism" and thus further entrenched policy-makers' avoidance of preventive measures; deepened both the reality of U.S. decline and its reactionary efforts to preserve its pre-eminent position; facilitated more assertiveness by rising powers who now champion their own "civilizational" models (thus strengthening the discourse of "the West" vs. "the Rest"); increased skepticism about the value of cooperating internationally; and decreased the financial resources available for international bodies (such as the WHO).

Daniel Drezner (2020) picks up on this thread, by arguing that when we apply an international relations lens to our contemporary world, COVID-19—unlike previous historical instances of pandemics—may not bring about *transformational* change. For Drezner, the pandemic could only bring about such transformation if it triggered new structural dynamics or discontinuities in key variables that shape the pattern of world politics, such as the distribution of power or economic interests. But it may be that factors beyond these material ones could shape our post-COVID world, particularly given our context of "crisis politics." Indeed, Drezner himself allows that the pandemic could have important ideational and "second-image" effects, either by challenging the hegemony of paradigms that value efficiency and the maximization of income, and/or by shifting countries away from populism and neo-liberalism. Similarly, Krebs acknowledges that there is always potential for the transformational opportunities inherent in crises to be seized by individuals, despite structures that seem to push in a contrary direction.

Building on this logic—which points to the potential of ideas and counter-narratives—we argue that the transition period out of deep crisis into a post-COVID world still offers opportunities to both rethink and recraft global governance solutions.

To begin, our current moment has included an acute sense of urgency, which we know from history has galvanized innovative governance design in the past. Furthermore, the key "rising powers" are still committed to the reform of international institutions, rather than their wholesale overthrow—a fact that is novel historically and that should be leveraged for positive change. Relatedly, the crisis has heightened the profile of non-Western actors whose empowerment can both help with generating new ideas and sharing the burden of providing for global public goods. Finally, there is widespread recognition among elites that avoiding another pandemic is in their interests *and* that any effective preventive action requires the cooperation of the broader population. This offers the possibility that global governance could be re-legitimized by ensuring that it works for the many, as well as the few.

Many scenarios for a post-COVID world are possible, including those with frightening implications—particularly if we jump from the "COVID frying pan into the climate fire" (Hepburn et al. 2020, 4). However, what we set out below are minimalist and maximalist scenarios for how global governance *could be improved* in a post-COVID world. They differ in terms of how extensively they seek to reconfigure global governance mechanisms, particularly in the service of enhancing the well-being of populations. More specifically, while the minimalist approach is primarily technocratic and aimed at system maintenance—similar to that in the wake of the financial crisis of 2008—the maximalist approach dares to acknowledge and explicitly work with the political dynamics that underpin global governance.

A Minimalist Vision

There are a variety of ways that global governance could be improved in the immediate term, through initiatives primarily aimed at the health and economic effects of the crisis. Under this approach, policy responses would draw upon existing institutions and appeal to the immediate interests of powerful states, but not significantly address global political, economic, and social imbalances. One of its core aims would be to ward off visible and latent tendencies towards deglobalization, and to assist those countries hardest hit by the pandemic with immediate economic and technical assistance.

In the economic realm, for example, we might see an international fiscal stimulus package coordinated by the G20, further upgrading the COVID line of credit of the International Monetary Fund (IMF), and to an even greater degree economic burden-sharing within regional organizations such as the European Union. The idea would be to focus on policy coordination to increase collective capacity, not the creation of new rules. The World Bank and regional development banks might engage in more intense collaboration on post-pandemic recovery, and individual countries might choose to surge bilateral development assistance to particularly hard-hit areas of the world. A ministerial conference of the World Trade Organization (WTO) might be organized to make sure protectionist measures do not, in future, apply to vital medical supplies.

Within the health field, we could see some modest reforms of WHO, including through the ongoing negotiations on a new "pandemic treaty", as well as new inter-agency mechanisms for improved early warning on infectious diseases with pandemic potential. A commission of experts might be struck—not unlike the International Panel on Climate Change—to report regularly on infectious disease, and to identify and disseminate best practices on strengthening health infrastructure and social policy, as well as the transportation and border policies that might be adopted in a future crisis. A multinational group of epidemiologists and public health specialists, perhaps with funding from a major foundation, could set out a blueprint for a permanent mechanism (building on the COVAX facility created during the pandemic) to ensure the equitable distribution of future vaccines. A Special Session of the UN General Assembly might be held to discuss the impact of COVID-19 and the need for greater preparation for future pandemics.[5]

Turning to the domain of peace and security, the UN Security Council might agree, under one of its rotating presidencies, to hold a thematic debate on infectious disease as a threat to international peace and security and agree to the creation of a "global health security coordinator" that could galvanize relevant actors across the UN and Bretton Woods system.[6] A special funding stream to support pandemic treatments in refugee camps might also be initiated, managed by the UN Refugee Agency (UNHCR). More political support from major powers might be mobilized to support ceasefires in conflict zones hard hit by pandemics like COVID-19, as called for by the UN Secretary-General in April 2020. And where the members of the Security Council remain deadlocked on responses to crises, regional security organizations might begin to draw on precedents from Africa in the early 1990s, in which bodies such as the Economic Community of West African States (ECOWAS) empowered its members to use force collectively to address safety challenges without prior authorization from the UN. Alternatively, in the face of Council paralysis, states with common security interests could independently create what international lawyers Oona Hathaway and Scott Shapiro (2020) have recently termed "global clubs." These groupings of states would share the burdens and costs of a variety of goods—for example, protection from cyberattacks—while denying the benefits to "bad actors."

Finally, in terms of the U.S.-China relationship, the two powers might agree to a form of global health *détente*, through which they would depoliticize WHO, increase its funding, and enable the organization to play its important functional roles.[7] More broadly, they could engage in forms of quiet diplomacy that could result in the creation of specific "hot lines" or crisis management tools—much like those that were developed between Washington and Moscow during the Cold War following the Cuban Missile Crisis. These efforts could better manage the rivalry between them and prevent disputes from escalating into military confrontation.

Overall, then, the minimalist vision is a concerted effort in "patch and repair," which would attempt to put the brakes on further deterioration of international cooperation. In fact, one of its primary tasks would be to prove, once again, that cooperation *can* sometimes work. But it would operate on the assumption that the underlying political and economic paradigms that has underpinned global governance are still appropriate and legitimate: they simply need renewed commitment, more creative policy options, and a willingness to implement. Above all, the minimalist approach would remain responsive rather than preventive in its orientation.

A Maximalist Vision

A maximalist approach to rethinking global governance would, primarily, acknowledge that governance is ultimately a political task. It would admit that there is not a single recipe for how best to achieve security and prosperity, but rather multiple views that require the hard work of compromise and reconciliation. It would therefore not only rely on the enlightened self-interest of powerful states to (grudgingly) accept isolated reforms, but also address the structural power asymmetries that have marked the post-1945 multilateral system.[8] In short, it would seek to elevate forms of solidarity and equity, not just as "nice to haves," but as crucial ingredients and core *interests* of those participating in global governance. Responding to the needs and aspirations of the disadvantaged, and their contestation of globalization in its current form, would certainly make such governance "messier" and more difficult. But by tackling grievance, rather than papering over it, the maximalist strategy could also make governance more just and sustainable.

This more ambitious path seeks to ensure that COVID-19 is an opportunity seized rather than an opportunity missed. What we sketch out here is a kind of "post-COVID settlement," aimed broadly at a more social-democratic world order that: (1) leverages governments' embrace of social policies during the pandemic, which would have been unthinkable prior to COVID-19; and (2) expands and directs

them across countries through productive processes of "policy transfer." It also seeks to build a representative governance architecture to
deliberate on these goals, and new mechanisms to finance them.

Although this maximalist vision might be described as pie in the
sky, its foundations are not entirely new; it relies on concepts, proposals, and debates that have been around for decades. Moreover, it
could be based initially on a renewed commitment to the realization
of the SDGs, which emerged from the most inclusive process of global
policy development yet attempted and which aspire to the creation of
a global partnership for sustainable development *everywhere* (not just
in the so-called Global South).

There are three broad dimensions to the maximalist approach.
The first—enhanced participation—seeks to *empower those states and
key non-state actors whose voices have been marginalized within global governance structures and processes.* Think of it as "enlarging the franchise"—
a maxim that could be applied to a variety of multilateral institutions.
For example, within the UN framework, this could entail the creation
of a UN parliamentary assembly, a more structured division of labour
between the UN and regional organizations, reform of the Security
Council's membership and working methods, and the granting of
a stronger policy-proposing role in matters of peace and security to
both the General Assembly and the UN Secretary-General. It could
also involve more concerted efforts to give key cities a place at the
table in decision-making on sustainable development and migration.
These steps will undoubtedly expose conflicting views and re-politi-
cize specific issues, particularly the liberal philosophy underpinning
contemporary globalization. But we believe that politics—far from
being the problem—are essential to addressing cleavages and recon-
ciling and aggregating different interests.

The second dimension—new instruments—recognizes that reform
of existing institutions is insufficient. We also need *new tools to facilitate
collective action in key economic, security, environmental, and social areas.*
Many proposals for new instruments and governance approaches
have already been hinted at in other chapters in this volume. One particular area of acute need is technology. The pandemic revealed all
too clearly why public authorities need accurate and timely data, both
to design good policy and to counteract damaging misinformation.
Yet, the incentives driving big tech companies remain at odds with
the public interest. Moreover, as our haphazard approach to governing the digital economy has only reinforced geopolitical divides, as

China, the United States, and the European Union each represent distinct technology systems—with incompatible norms, regulatory regimes, and corporate and state interests (Medhora and Owen 2020). Finally, we have no equitable or effective governance mechanisms for the key driver of the digital economy—intellectual property—and nor have we tackled the problem of tax arbitrage by multinationals. For all these reasons, Rohinton Medhora and Taylor Owen call for a big and bold governance intervention—a "digital Bretton Woods"—aimed at addressing the clear need for data governance and for mechanisms to manage the digital and intangible economy.

Another obvious domain is the governance of global health itself, where a new framing of the problem is urgently required. Rather than reinforcing the language of security—which entails a strategy of focusing primarily on the threat of pandemics—developed countries could acknowledge that the developing world has many other pressing health priorities, some of which they prioritize ahead of viruses such as COVID-19. For its part, the developing world could leverage this particular moment, when rich countries "are listening," to argue for a transformation of the global health discussion, where notions of human rights and solidarity, rather than security, are paramount and where more sizeable resources (from private actors as well as governments) are transferred to produce better and more sustainable health structures and outcomes.

These technology and health proposals point to the final dimension of our maximalist vision: the *need for new resources to support global policy making in security and sustainable development*. Without new sources of funding—which could come from corporate profits, financial transactions, arms sales, and the like—new global governance proposals will remain just that: *proposals*. Furthermore, without a process to move from revenue raising to revenue distribution, there is a risk that larger markets will keep most of the funds from taxation.

Conclusion

Is the maximalist approach possible? How do we get there? Over the years, many proposals have been made to reform or transform global governance. Although we do not think the maximalist scenario is the most likely one, we do believe it remains feasible as piecemeal solutions do not address the fundamental global challenges. One of the main obstacles is the potential opposition of today's two great powers and/or the politicization of governance that stems from their rivalry. Nonetheless, there are two sources of optimism. First, while the self-exclusion of the United States from the League of Nations fatally undermined it in the inter-war period, we also know that the UN Charter was only signed by 51 countries in 1945, before the rest of the world joined them. Second, close study of the early Cold War shows that bipolarity itself was not the driver of superpower rivalry, but rather a dynamic of mistrust that intensified as the United States and Soviet Union clashed over questions such as war reparations and the division of Germany. If smart diplomacy, both official and unofficial, can work today to pre-emptively build channels of communication and identify areas for constructive collaboration, a divided world and weak global governance may not be preordained.

Notes

1. The statement is available at https://g20.org/en/media/Documents/G20_Extraordinary%20G20%20Leaders'%20Summit_Statement_EN%20(3).pdf.
2. We credit this phrase to our fellow political scientist, Professor Janice Stein.
3. Most notably, this resolution took the significant step of declaring the pandemic a threat to international peace and security. See the details of the resolution at https://www.un.org/press/en/2014/sc11566.doc.htm.
4. Paul Romer, 2004, quoted by Jack Rosenthal, "A Terrible Thing to Waste," *The New York Times,* July 31, 2009, https://www.nytimes.com/2009/08/02/magazine/02FOB-onlanguage-t.html.
5. In fact, as this book was going to press, the UN General Assembly held such a debate during its 78th Session, and on 20 September 2023 issued a Political Declaration on Pandemic Preparedness and Response.
6. This is one proposal that emerged from the Council on Foreign Relations Taskforce on Pandemic Preparedness and Lessons from COVID-19. The report is available at https://www.cfr.org/report/pandemic-preparedness-lessons-COVID-19/.
7. We would like to thank colleague and global health specialist David Fidler for suggesting this idea.
8. For example, within the IMF, the United States has over 16 percent of the voting power while China has only 6 percent; the G7 group of advanced economies, which account for roughly 30 percent of world output, have over 40 percent of the voting power.

References

Acharya, Amitav. 2018. "Multilateralism and the Changing World Order." In *The Oxford Handbook of the United Nations,* 2nd ed., edited by Thomas G. Weiss and Sam Daws, 781–796. Oxford: Oxford University Press.

Berman, Sheri. 2020. "Crises Only Sometimes Lead to Change. Here's Why." *Foreign Policy,* July 4, 2020. https://foreignpolicy.com/2020/07/04/coronavirus-crisis- turning-point-change/.

Drezner, Daniel. 2020. "The Song Remains the Same: International Relations After COVID-19." *International Organization* 74 (S1): E18–E35. https://doi:10.1017/S0020818320000387.

Guterres, António. 2020. "Remarks to the Security Council on the COVID-19 Pandemic." United Nations Secretary-General. April 9, 2020. https://www.un.org/sg/en/content/sg/speeches/2020-04-09/remarks-security-council-covid-19-pandemic.

Haass, Richard. 2020. "The Pandemic Will Accelerate History Rather than Reshape It: Not Every Crisis Is a Turning Point." *Foreign Affairs*, April 7, 2020. https://www.foreignaffairs.com/articles/united-states/2020-04-07/pandemic-will-accelerate-history-rather-reshape-it.

Hale, Thomas, and David Held, eds. 2017. *Beyond Gridlock*. Cambridge: Polity Press.

Hathaway, Oona, and Scott J. Shapiro. 2020. "Welcome to the Post-Leader World." *Foreign Policy*, July 4, 2020. https://foreignpolicy.com/2020/07/04/after-hegemony/.

Hepburn, Cameron, Brian O'Callaghan, Nicholas Stern, Joseph Stiglitz, and Dimitri Zenghelis. 2020. "Will COVID-19 Fiscal Recovery Packages Accelerate or Retard Progress on Climate Change?" *Oxford Review of Economic Policy* 36 (S1): S359–S381. https://doi.org/10.1093/oxrep/graa015.

Huang, Yanzhong. 2021. "Why the World Lost to the Pandemic: Politics and Security Fears Crippled the Collective Response." *Foreign Affairs*, January 28, 2021. https://www.foreignaffairs.com/articles/united-states/2021-01-28/why-world-lost-pandemic#author-info.

Kaplan, Robert D. 2020. "Coronavirus Ushers in the Globalization We Were Afraid Of." *Bloomberg*, May 20, 2020. https://www.bloomberg.com/opinion/articles/2020-03-20/coronavirus-ushers-in-the-globalization-we-were-afraid-of.

Krebs, Ronald R. 2015. *Narrative and the Making of US National Security*. Cambridge: Cambridge University Press.

Lecler, Romain. 2020. "Le Covid-19 met au jour toute une série de phénomènes associés à la mondialisation." *Le Monde*, March 6, 2020. https://www.lemonde.fr/idees/article/2020/03/06/le-covid-19-met-au-jour-toute-une-serie-de-phenomenes-associes-a-la-mondialisation_6032092_3232.html.

Louis, Marieke. 2020. "L'OMS dans le maelstrom du Covid-19 : Entretien avec Auriane Guilbaud. " *La vie des idées*, April 13, 2020. https://laviedesidees.fr/L-OMS-dans-le-maelstrom-du-covid-19.html.

McNamara, Kathleen R., and Abraham L. Newman. 2020. "The Big Reveal: COVID-19 and Globalization's Great Transformations." *International Organization* 74 (S1): E59–E77. https:// doi:10.1017/S0020818320000387.

Medhora, Rohinton P., and Taylor Owen. 2020. "A Post-COVID-19 Digital Bretton Woods." *Project Syndicate*, April 17, 2020. https://www.project-syndicate.org/onpoint/digital-bretton-woods-new-global-governance-

model-by-rohinton-p-medhora-and-taylor-owen-2020-04?barrier=
accesspaylog.

Munich Security Conference (MSC). 2020. "Polypandemic." Munich Security
Report Special Edition on Development, Fragility, and Conflict in
the Era of Covid-19. November 2020. https://securityconference.org/
assets/02_Dokumente/01_Publikationen/201104_MSC_Polypandemic_
EN.pdf.

Summers, Lawrence. 2020. "Covid-19 Looks Like a Hinge in History." *Foreign
Affairs*, April 7, 2020. https://www.ft.com/content/de643ae8-9527-11ea-
899a-f62a20d54625.

Trudeau, Justin. 2020. "Extraordinary G20 Leaders' Summit Statement on
COVID-19." Prime Minister of Canada, Government of Canada (web-
site). March 26, 2020. https://pm.gc.ca/en/news/statements/2020/03/26/
extraordinary-g20-leaders-summit-statement-covid-19.

United Nations. 2014. "Global Governance and Global Rules for Development
in the Post-2015 Era." Committee for Development Policy. June 2014.
https://www.un.org/development/desa/dpad/wp-content/uploads/
sites/45/publication/2014-cdp-policy.pdf.

United Nations. 2020. "External Finance and Inclusive Growth." Discussion
notes from the United Nations' High Level Event on Financing for
Development in the Era of COVID-19 and Beyond, convened by
Canada, Jamaica, and the Secretary-General on May 28, 2020. https://
www.un.org/sites/un2.un.org/files/2020/05/discussion_note_3-private_
sector_creditors-_hle_ffd_covid-5-25-20.pdf.

Vilmer, Jean-Baptiste Jeangène. 2020. "Il n'y aura pas de monde après."
Politique internationale 168 (Summer 2020): 131–156. https://politiquein-
ternationale.com/revue/n168/article/il-ny-aura-pas-de-monde-dapres.

World Bank. 2020. *Macro Poverty Outlook: Country-by-Country Analysis and
Projections for the Developing World*. Washington D.C.: World Bank.
https://www.worldbank.org/en/publication/macro-poverty-outlook.

CHAPTER 2

Global Health

Laurence Monnais, Ryoa Chung,
Pierre-Marie David, and Thomas Druetz

After the initial wave of shock, COVID-19 gave way to a proliferation of philanthro-capitalist interests "investing in health" and a return to health isolationism, saturated with the promises of biomedical techno-solutionism. Yet the pandemic is seemingly the perfect context for rethinking global health. In this chapter, we propose a *counter-reform* of global health and—in particular—of global *public health*, by examining the power dynamics that influence the field of health. In speaking of "counter-reform," we are promoting an alternative to the increasingly enormous injection of private funds into health care and to technological innovations likely to increase inequalities in this field. We use the term "public health" to emphasize the importance of a political space for responses based on collective prevention and the promotion of population health.

Global health is a multidisciplinary field that looks at health as the result of historical forces and processes that transcend national borders and involve actors from various spheres of human activity. Global health, which—in its purpose and practice—aims to improve population health by reducing injustice, encompasses the political, economic, social, environmental, and epidemiological aspects of health concerns at a time of accelerating globalization. Although it is the product of the international health initiatives that emerged from nineteenth-century colonial empires, it is unique in that it sees health first and foremost as an issue of equity.

The Pandemic—Overlooking and Revealing Inequalities

The SARS-CoV-2 coronavirus—first identified in the Chinese mega-city of Wuhan in November 2019—led to half the world's population in over 90 countries going into lockdown on 1 April 2020. This measure—a long-standing practice but implemented on a scale unprecedented in the history of pandemics—struck a chord because of the speed with which states invoked its application. Hundreds of millions of people were confined to their homes; national economies were "on hold," and countries withdrew into themselves, within once-again tight borders. This threefold approach seems paradoxical given that human and commercial mobility has accelerated over the last 30 years.

Generalized lockdowns form part of so-called "preparedness policies" (David and Le Dévédec 2019), which began in the 1990s and flourished in the wake of the 11 September 2001 attacks and the 2003 severe acute respiratory syndrome (SARS) epidemic as a result of an obsession with security that combined two fears: of terrorism and the use of biological weapons. What preparedness means in the context of a potential pandemic is the introduction of "physical distancing" measures that have worked in the past, notably during the 1918–1919 H1N1 influenza pandemic (Markel et al. 2006). These measures aim to contain the disease until "pharmaceutical solutions," such as drugs or vaccines, are developed.

These prescriptive measures were formalized without regard to the political, economic, sociocultural, or even healthcare contexts. The political decision to introduce these measures in 2020 was based on real-time morbidity and mortality statistics, as well as on outbreak projections—some of them catastrophic—that were developed using sophisticated mathematical models of logarithmic diffusion but ill-suited to the course of an unknown and versatile pathogen that evolves according to biological, societal, individual, and even collective responses.

Furthermore, preparedness policies were imposed on hospital-centric healthcare systems that were already under stress, chronically underfunded and under-equipped, in response to policies of austerity aimed at improving efficiency and even ensuring profitability. As a result, "flattening the curve" was key to avoid saturating intensive care units. This approach underlined the on-going erasure of public health as an institutionalized field of intervention, that educates and promotes good collective health (Monnais 2020). Conversely, lockdowns are a response guided by a technical and biomedical vision that makes medical resources the gold standard of any response, the only way to avoid a double disaster—clinical (too many hospitalized patients) and statistical (too many deaths).

Although this radical containment model spread like wildfire in a matter of weeks, not all governments supported it. Other collective virus-protection methods were implemented—some successfully. The screening–tracking–isolation approach a number of Asian countries (e.g., South Korea, Taiwan, Vietnam, Thailand) adopted, led by recent viral experiments, allowed them to circumscribe containment areas rapidly. Several countries relied on the early use of masks— which they had stockpiled and made widely available—and on practical, benevolent education on the benefits of physical distancing for the common good (e.g., New Zealand and Portugal).

COVID-19 also thwarted predictions of contamination of the "North" by the "South." As one of the world's leading economic powers, China is not part of the South—a Global South that is difficult to define. Nevertheless, it remains one of the countries of the nineteenth century's so-called "Asia, the cradle of cholera"—of SARS and avian flu—the origin of persistent claims of a developing, non-Western, pathogenic space, which have played on the astonishing short-sightedness of political and public health authorities in European and North American countries. As late as February 2020, some governments believed that the West would avoid the wave or, at the very least, easily cope with this "flu."

Lastly, the coronavirus not only affected countries in a disproportionate way, but it also targeted specific communities. These transnational groups were vulnerable to both the pathogen and to the impacts of the measures implemented to stop its spread, the latter emphasizing the individual and their responsibility rather than their actual ability to isolate. These groups turned out to be minorities in their experience: refugees, prisoners, disadvantaged ethnic minorities, unhoused people, those subject to domestic violence, people with substance-use disorders, seniors in long-term care homes, and the largely female, immigrant, low-skilled, and underpaid staff working with them.

The SARS-CoV-2 experience revealed not only how *life* is fetishized, but also the inequality of *lives* (Fassin 2018). It has forced us to re-examine global health paradigms. The "down-up" spread of homemade face coverings, which began in March 2020 in various public spaces where health authorities have long resisted recommending they be worn, citing their ineffectiveness—even dangerousness—and the fact that they had no foothold in the culture, suggests that the obliviousness towards public health may be reversible. For a time at least, the use of masks was an encouraging sign of supportive, enlightened and—above all—pragmatic citizen participation in fair and effective prevention, resistant to social erasure in the face of the market.

Vulnerability, Systemic Injustice, and the Right to Health Care

The pandemic showed the decisive role social inequalities play in population health on a national and global scale. Excluding the emergency measures that accompanied it, which obscured the reality and impacts of these inequalities, COVID-19 revealed the need to strengthen forms of social protection, combat discrimination, and prioritize the reduction of socioeconomic precarity and vulnerability to improve health. While these inequalities are not new, the pandemic highlighted the failings of societies where they appear to be systemic. In this respect, the current moment is the perfect opportunity to take stock of failures in terms of the right to health, social justice, and the international community's responsibility to improve health.

The genesis of modern discourse on the right to health as a fundamental right can be traced back to the birth of the Red Cross and the emergence of international humanitarian law at the end of the nineteenth century. While we should be wary of viewing the highly political history of the United Nations (UN) model of post-1945 international relations through rose-tinted glasses, it is important to remember that this right is an integral part of the mission of the World Health Organization (WHO) (1948 Constitution, section 25). Philosophically, the right to health can be seen as a fundamental right (i.e., a prerequisite for the exercise of all other rights)—hence the centrality of universal health coverage. In other words, the right to health can be understood as effectively exercising an "ability to be healthy" (Sen 2002). This approach requires us to consider a country's subjective and objective dimensions and how they vary over time and according to the actors involved.

However, the way we think about human rights—and the institutions and conventions that claim them—is part of a Western history which, despite its universalist aspirations, is shaped by profound violence and injustice. This Western-inspired model is regularly confronted with forms of cultural pluralism and a polysemy of the very notion of health that cannot be satisfied with a biomedical response, leading to veiled epistemic injustices that accentuate hierarchies in the production of health knowledge.

Epistemic injustice (Fricker 2007) refers to morally arbitrary inequalities that affect both individuals and knowledge. The complex relationship between knowledge and power gives rise to inequalities of status between individuals considered to be legitimate producers of knowledge. Because of prejudice and discrimination, some individuals or social groups suffer from a lack of credibility. Certain categories of testimony or interpretations of the world are declared unintelligible or are denigrated by individuals or groups in a position of epistemic authority, who impose their own cognitive resources as the dominant paradigm.

Whatever the justification, the right to health is not a given: defended out of moral conviction by some and exploited by others, it is moored to questions of equity and social justice—a link that is highlighted in discussions on the social determinants of health, which emphasizes the critical importance of policies for distributing resources within a society in order to ensure good collective health. While systematic lockdowns ignore both upstream inequalities and their potential downstream exacerbation, the pandemic quickly revealed the impact of class, gender, and racial inequalities—as well as disability and age-related vulnerabilities—on the ability of individuals and communities to avoid getting sick and cope with its economic impacts.

These structural vulnerabilities (Chung and Hunt 2012) must not be "essentialized," but rather analyzed in terms of context (Ahmad et al. 2020). For example, ageism—which, under the guise of benevolent paternalism—gave rise to excessive constraints imposed on the elderly, while the pandemic revealed the extent to which their interests had been neglected. COVID-19 shone a harsh light on cases of physical and psychological neglect in some care facilities—both in Quebec and elsewhere—that were exacerbated by visiting bans during lockdowns. While over 80 percent of official deaths caused by COVID-19 occurred in long-term care facilities or private seniors' residences, the Institut national de santé publique du Québec found that a lack of political representation for seniors in many societies, which view them as an economic burden has undoubtedly helped intensify their vulnerability.

This marginalization, discrimination, and social hierarchy help cement structural injustices on a local and global scale. These injustices also call into question the neoliberal practices that produce them: a stratified division of labour and standards that differ by social class, which lead to some suffering virtually no harm, while others are seen as both essential and interchangeable workers (e.g., undocumented caregivers or seasonal labourers). The duty to correct these injustices falls to the international community, but it also requires a renewed awareness of the abysmal inequalities that exist between those who enjoy a quality of life that drains all resources and those who are brutally deprived of it.

In light of the plight of the 1 percent of the world's population who are refugees or stateless, we have to agree with Hannah Arendt that "the right to have rights" is a critical precondition for protecting human dignity (1966, 296–297). The human right to health is a moral duty incumbent on the international community, and it goes above and beyond the criteria of citizenship. Consequently, global health governance cannot be confined to controlling infectious diseases. The pandemic forces us to rethink risk-sharing; it gives us an opportunity to reprioritize the notion of a "shared destiny," which requires ethical and equitable cooperation. Rhetorical posturing aside, the call for simple discretionary charity must lead to a duty to rectify historical wrongs and structural injustices that entail a more equitable redistribution of resources, in particular to support genuine global health governance.

Strengthening the Importance of People and Their Work

A number of decision-makers, experts, and commentators are advocating for increasingly powerful technological solutions to improve people's health. Mobile applications and drones are being added to an array of miracle pills and artificial intelligence's intensive megadata exploitation. In this reductionist perspective, the future of global health care would be hyper-technological, erasing not only the individual and collective experience of health and illness but also human work, which lies at the very core of health inequalities and their reduction.

Technology is helping redefine ways of acting according to needs; our relationship with technology is the subject of highly optimistic or—conversely—highly pessimistic predictions and, to a lesser extent, realistic criticism, particularly of how technology enables well-known power dynamics involving cross-discriminations of gender, race, and class to be replayed. It is essential to question the importance of bio-medical technological advances, but we must remember that behind every syringe is an experienced and skilled "hand." Furthermore, the coronavirus pandemic has shown that this hand is key to understanding why technological tools (e.g., serological tests, tracking applications) are missing, and also why many caregivers—women caregivers in particular—become contaminated.

Lockdowns have highlighted the relevance—or even necessity—of certain types of human work that have been forgotten, devalued, or downplayed, including in the healthcare sector. While resuscitation care in hospitals must be able to rely on sophisticated machines, it exists first and foremost on the basis of duly trained and available personnel. At the same time, we have seen that the least-qualified healthcare workers, offering front-line care in often extreme conditions, have been at least as exposed to the virus as hospital doctors. The response, or absence, of orderlies, stretcher-bearers, and maintenance workers has shown that healthcare systems are truly that—*systems*—(i.e., interdependent spaces within which each individual is critical for the whole to function), and it has highlighted long-invisible value chains in the production of care.

Human work must once again become something that is valued, which is posed in terms other than those of victimization or heroization—two processes that fuel a martial approach, a so-called "war on the virus" that must be won, but above all that prevent any debate on the place of these workers in the political and public arenas and that undermine their fair recognition, including pay. In the context of healthcare systems and global medical treatment, we need to ask ourselves what an acceptable pay gap would look like, whether between doctors and orderlies or between international and local staff. The occasional bonuses several countries offer to both orderlies and doctors do not resolve this issue.

While healthcare systems depend on a wide range of care workers with interrelated skills and experience, it is also critical to question these workers' role in decision-making processes, including in the area of prevention. Since the 1990s, healthcare organizations have been run by managers and examined by consultancy firms, whose aim is to rationalize services by focusing more on measurement than meaning. Alongside this neoliberal logic that subjects health care to predominantly managerial and accounting reasoning, intersectoral working committees — in this case both interprofessional and interdisciplinary — must have their say.

Calling for the democratization of healthcare organizations also highlights the international asymmetries that exist in how healthcare workers are used. Because of the high demand for staff, the most industrialized countries are looking to countries in the South for qualified workers (often in the form of "acting as"), which in effect means downgrading. Without professional recognition or pay, these jobs deepen existing hierarchies. They also leave countries with a shortage of healthcare workers and amplify geographical inequalities in access to care.

A corollary of this democratization is another effort at horizontalization. Vertical, hierarchical operation has often been favoured as a means of improving the efficiency of healthcare systems and care. However, recognizing the social value of this type of work means that those who operate healthcare systems (i.e., professionals, ordinary citizens, volunteers, and caregivers) can establish care and meaning in their communities in a more horizontal way. For example, the proposal for a "community health corps," — a "set of workers who could support those in need while maintaining collective health and building genuine solidarity" (Gonsalves and Kapczynski 2020) — asserts that a new approach to care that is centred on a commitment to providing universal services based on need is possible. In addition to doing the tracing work too quickly handed over to technological applications, these workers could ensure that the families involved have the material and social resources needed to quarantine themselves, or that any "non-serious" COVID-19 cases are followed up on to detect any chronic symptoms. By extension, we are advocating a return to *pragmatic*, grassroots public health care that is based on the solidarity of a range of stakeholders working to improve daily life and the collective good.

From this point of view, global health needs to acknowledge the implicit hierarchy of its knowledge and rectify certain asymmetries in its choice of referents and models. In contrast to the situation in Europe and North America, in several West African and Southeast Asian countries, the human worker — in the guise of community health workers, sometimes volunteers — was the one who sounded the alarm early about symptomatic individuals and traced their contacts by going door to door in record time. Based on previous experience (e.g., with Ebola in Nigeria, and SARS and avian flu in Vietnam), we now understand that while this approach was certainly led, at the time, by public health authorities, it was not highly technological and was able to preserve people's fundamental rights.

In the face of the governance of numbers and technologies, reaffirming the right to work in general (Supiot 2015)—more specifically that of healthcare workers—rather than seeking to make it more flexible, or even subject to the imperatives of trade or intellectual property, is a condition for exercising fundamental rights, which includes the right to health. These rights, which led to the creation of founding institutions (the International Labour Organization in 1919, the WHO in 1948) that assert their superiority over force—military in the past and economic in the present—must, above all, underpin a new ethic of international relations and prescribe a counter-reform of global health, in particular its governance. While the "one health" paradigm—an integrated approach to human, animal, and environmental health—means considering health *beyond* the human, the latter must remain at the heart of the global health project as a value, a task, and a goal that give it meaning and that can in no way be reduced to an adjustment variable for technological promises.

Counter-Reforming Global Health Governance

With the rapid spread of COVID-19, global health governance experienced a dual phenomenon. First, countries were asked to take extraordinary measures to protect their people. There has been a kind of return to the sovereign state, with control mechanisms to ensure that collective well-being is deployed. This movement is a revival of *res publica*, and even a return to the legitimacy of state bodies. However, it is also based on a state reflex of looking inward "for the good of the nation," and it is more often a matter of biosecurity than of emancipation, of populism than of effective protection.

Second, we are witnessing a crisis in the international health structure. As the only organization with a mandate to improve the health of the world's population, the WHO is now a political arena with clashing ideologies—the shock exit of the United States in July 2020 being a perfect example—rather than a multilateral action-oriented mechanism guided by consultation and the pooling of expertise.

Several successive epidemics of (re)emerging diseases (e.g., SARS, Ebola, H1N1, Zika) have peaked the institution's internal tensions and revealed its three flaws: funding, governance, and operations.

Chronic underfunding by Member States forces the WHO to turn to non-state backers, chief among them the Bill & Melinda Gates Foundation, to ensure that its projects are carried out, making it vulnerable to private interests. Submitting to competitive and biomedical requirements—based in ideology—stems from a vision of health care as a "return on investment." It increases the role of the audit and consultancy industry, adding to an already imposing bureaucracy, and leads to an obsession with performance and quantified accountability. This not only hampers the smooth operation of global health care, but also highlights the fact that treatment is done in fits and starts, at the whim of volatile priorities that are detached from complex epidemiological realities and social injustices. In a sort of vicious circle that contributes to nation-states resigning and the welfare state declining, this submission increases major powers' resistance to granting the WHO excessively restrictive powers, particularly in times of health crises, which undermines the institution's technical and political authority and—by extension—its ability to fulfill its mandate.

The visible erosion of multilateralism and the growing weight of philanthro-capitalism (Birn, Pillay, and Holtz 2017) reinforce each other and revive—in the context of the pandemic—a "realistic" view of the international order, centred on countries and their (bio)securitization, and where national interest takes precedence over international solidarity. Contributing to exposing powers rather than unifying them in a collective response, SARS-CoV-2 carries in its wake a "privatized biomedicalization" of health care that operates in silos— one healthcare problem at a time—avoided or taken care of by segmented actors within the framework of national borders that do not govern the outcome of the pandemic (Druetz 2018). The availability of medical supplies and the terms of access to vaccines, which require our own pandemic-response tools to be simultaneously offshored and financialized, are perfect examples of these politically based ethical tensions that are bearers of new health and social inequalities—both endogenous and transnational—within which competition prevails over solidarity.

At a time when the pandemic has highlighted the need for multilateral prevention mechanisms, and when Member States are in the process of negotiating a new legal instrument for pandemic preparedness and response, the WHO must not only re-establish its legitimacy and neutrality, but also renew its political ambitions in terms of the right to health and health justice. It will have to go beyond the provisions of the International Health Regulations, which were amended in 2005 in the wake of SARS, and outline a series of duties for WHO Member States, including the duty to declare the presence of infectious diseases likely to pose a risk to supranational health. The need for transparency and a code of ethics, as well as a discussion on the involvement of private interests (and not simply of private funds), are among the work the WHO must do toward counter-reform, which would consist of making its financing and operating methods more independent and even endowing it with more binding powers vis-à-vis Member States. Vital tools for tangibly improving international health governance include creating a body for settling political disputes, revising its legal and budgetary framework, and establishing technical criteria approved prior to decision-making.

In addition, one of the WHO's main saving graces may be to adopt a concept of global health that is not the "health of others;" it must decompartmentalize the "them" from the "us" both between and within countries—a process that begun timidly with the recognition of universal Sustainable Development Goals (2015). Committed to a decolonial project (Eichbaum et al. 2020), it will need to recognize and draw on local expertise from vulnerable communities and developing countries to shed the weighty dual heritage of colonial medicine and international health, of a humanitarian—if not civilizational—duty that gives it the right to intervene in the "lives of the South" to foster development (Packard 2016).

Ethical sharing of scientific knowledge on an equal footing would not only unearth expertise that has been suppressed—due to a lack of professional status or a history of oppression (Cormak and Paine 2020)—but would also give pride of place to experiential knowledge, that of community workers, field epidemiologists, mothers, Elders, activists, associative groups, and patients. By deploying a more inclusive and collaborative form of governance that calls on a community of global health experts "beyond borders"—mixed and mobile (Ebikeme 2020)—it can formulate contextualized and sensitive recommendations and review universal recommendations, as well as advocate for measures to reduce infectious risks rather than a quest for zero risk, for example, as in the precursory case of the UNAIDS program (1995) in its fight against HIV/AIDS.

In other words, good global health governance requires a supranational governing body that prioritizes safety and preparedness in its multi-sectoral effort to obtain a right to health—both individual and collective—independent of market logics and imperatives, to strengthen the capacity of both public health systems and truly global public health to act. In view of the obvious failures of both isolationist reflexes and neoliberal strategies, the WHO has—more than ever—a role to play in overcoming the challenges of a global health system that must promote population health through concerted, ambitious, and binding mechanisms.

Conclusion

The global health counter-reform we propose involves three collective processes: (1) defending a right to health that supports a form of social justice that is neither a duty, nor a (return on) investment, nor a utopian quest, but rather a responsibility that takes structural and epistemic injustices seriously; (2) prioritizing the person—rather than the number or the machine—which fits into inclusive and equitable community health systems, forgetting neither work and its fair valuation nor the plural experience of the field; and (3) overhauling global health governance, including reappropriating (and deprivatizing) existing international bodies and transforming ways of thinking about transnational dialogue beyond the imperatives of the market and the pitfalls of globalization. This counter-reform postulates a triple necessity upstream of crisis management and the anticipation of infectious risks: the demedicalization of health care, the transformation of the unbridled, chimerical race for technological innovation, and the liberation and decolonization of thought patterns that subordinate a South to an outdated North.

References

Ahmad, Ayesha, Ryoa Chung, Lisa Eckenwiler, Agomoni Ganguli-Mitra, Matthew Hunt, Rebecca Richards, Yashar Saghai, Lisa Schwartz, Jackie Leach Scully, and Verina Wild. 2020. "What Does It Mean to Be Made Vulnerable in the Era of COVID 19?" *The Lancet* 395, no. 10235 (May): 1481–1482.

Arendt, Hannah. 1966. *The Origins of Totalitarianism*. New York: Harcourt: Brace & World.

Birn, Anne-Emmanuelle, Yogan Pillay, and Timothy H. Holtz. 2017. *Textbook of Global Health*. 4th ed. Oxford: Oxford University Press.

Chung, Ryoa, and Matthew R. Hunt. 2012. "Justice and Health Inequalities in Humanitarian Crises: Structured Health Vulnerabilities and Natural Disaster." In *Health Inequalities and Global Justice*, edited by Patti Tamara Lenard and Christine Straehle, 197–212. Edinburgh: Edinburgh University Press.

Cormak, Donna, and Sarah-Jane Paine. 2020. "Dear Epidemiology: A Letter from Two Māori Researchers." *The Pantograph Punch*, May 15, 2020. https://pantograph-punch.com/posts/dear-epidemiology.

David, Pierre-Marie, and Nicolas Le Dévédec. 2019. "Preparedness for the Next Epidemic: Health and Political Issues of an Emerging Paradigm." *Critical Public Health* 29 (3): 363–369. https://doi.org/10.1080/09581596.2018.1447646.

Druetz, Thomas. 2018. "Integrated Primary Health Care in Low- and Middle-Income Countries: A Double Challenge." *BMC Medical Ethics* 19, no. S1: 48.

Ebikeme, Charles. 2020. "Expertise, Coronavirus, and the New Normal." *Think Global Health*, April 28, 2020. https://www.thinkglobalhealth.org/article/expertise-coronavirus-and-new-normal.

Eichbaum, Quentin G., Lisa V. Adams, Jessica Evert, Ming-Jung Ho, Innocent A. Semali, and Susan C. van Schalkwyk. 2020. "Decolonizing Global Health Education: Rethinking Institutional Partnerships and Approaches." *Academic Medicine* 96, no. 3 (March): 329–335. https://doi.org/10.1097/ACM.0000000000003473.

Fassin, Didier. 2018. *La vie. Mode d'emploi critique*. Paris: Éditions du Seuil.

Fricker, Miranda. 2007. *Epistemic Injustice. Power and the Ethics of Knowing*. Oxford: Oxford University Press.

Gonsalves, Gregg, and Amy Kapczynski. 2020. "The New Politics of Care." *The Boston Review. A Political and Literary Forum*, April 27, 2020. http://bostonreview.net/politics/gregg-gonsalves-amy-kapczynski-new-politics-care.

Institut national de santé publique du Québec. 2021. "Données COVID-19 — Comparaisons provinciales et internationales." Last modified March 12, 2021. https://www.inspq.qc.ca/covid-19/donnees/comparaisons.

Markel, Howard, Alexandra M. Stern, Alexander Navarro, Joseph R. Michalsen, Arnold S. Monto, and Cleto DiGiovanni. 2006. "Non-Pharmaceutical Influenza Mitigation Strategies, US Communities, 1918–1920 Pandemic." *Emerging Infectious Diseases* 12, no. 12 (December): 1961–1964. https://dx.doi.org/10.3201/eid1212.060506.

Monnais, Laurence. 2020. "Covid-19 ou l'indigence de la santé publique démasquée." *Analyse Opinion Critique (AOC)*, March 18, 2020. https://aoc.media/analyse/2020/03/17/covid-19-ou-lindigence-de-la-sante-publique-demasquee/.

Packard, Randall M. 2016. *A History of Global Health: Interventions into the Lives of Other Peoples*. Baltimore: Johns Hopkins University Press.

Sen, Amartya. 2015. "Why Health Equity?" *Health Economics* 11, no. 2 (December): 659–666.

Supiot, Alain. 2015. *Le gouvernance par les nombres*. Paris: Fayard.

CHAPTER 3

The Global Economy

Peter Dietsch, Vincent Arel-Bundock, Mark R. Brawley,
Allison Christians, Juliet Johnson, Krzysztof Pelc, and Ari Van Assche

We often only realize what we take for granted once it is no longer there. When COVID-19 struck in early 2020, life as we knew it came to a standstill. Whereas the public health measures have, for the most part, been lifted now, the economic repercussions will be felt for years to come. Workers were still slow to re-enter the labour market, especially in some sectors such as tourism and restaurants; both firms and governments will come out of the crisis with even higher levels of debt. Disruptions risk being particularly profound for transnational economic relations, where the virus has and will continue to upset delicate equilibria, and potentially even the way we organize our international economic institutions.

Alarm bells were initially rung over global trade, with merchandise trade dropping 18.5 percent in the second quarter of 2020 as compared to the same period in 2019, and with goods shortages due to supply chain bottlenecks dominating the headlines in the second half of 2021. In other key areas, such as fiscal and monetary policy, the challenges have become increasingly apparent over time. Governments spent, and rightly so, to support individuals and ailing businesses at the height of the crisis, but they had to borrow heavily in order to do so. How will international sovereign debt markets react to this enormous public debt in the medium term? How might central banks act in order to mitigate the historic economic slump we witnessed in the immediate aftermath of the crisis, and what trade-offs are involved in their choices? Most importantly, how can we contain crisis-induced socioeconomic inequalities and their political ramifications?

The goal of this chapter is to explore the major challenges arising from COVID-19 for trade, fiscal, and monetary policy, and to suggest policy responses to meet these challenges. We analyze the international political economy of the COVID-19 crisis in three temporal stages: emergency, recovery, and aftermath. In the *emergency phase*, public health considerations dictated public policy. As countries decided to prioritize economic considerations over health considerations, whether this shift was warranted or not, they put themselves in the *economic recovery phase*. Finally, in the *aftermath phase*, decision-makers need to take stock and consider more fundamental policy reforms to address the systemic weaknesses revealed by the crisis. Chief among these weaknesses, in our view, is the risk that crisis responses may exacerbate socioeconomic inequalities both within and between countries.

As a general rule, the more *temporally removed* from the emergency phase, the more leeway there will be for productively restructuring economic institutions. At the same time, as the immediate crisis recedes, policy makers may feel less pressure to act, and there is bound to be significant disagreement about next steps among both polities and governments. The capacity to effectively respond to the crisis economically will depend not only on short-term crisis management, but also on the ability of governments to anticipate unintended medium- and long-term side effects of their policies and actively cooperate to mitigate them even when the decisions required are not always popular.

The Emergency Phase

In order to understand subsequent national and multilateral policy reactions, we need to consider the dynamics set in motion during the height of the public health crisis. In particular, what characteristics of this crisis potentially set it apart from past crises?

Start with *international trade*. Once we look beyond the staggering decline in cross-border trade, two features distinguish this crisis from past ones: (1) the export restrictions that many states imposed on medical equipment; and (2) the widespread denunciation of global value chains through which multinational enterprises and their suppliers organize their production across several countries. The reasons are clear-cut. The rapid spread of the pandemic in the first quarter of 2020 led to an unanticipated, severe, and synchronized spike in the demand for medical equipment across the globe. Some 80 exporting countries reacted to the demand surge by restricting overseas sales of medical equipment. Other countries blamed structural flaws in global supply chains for local shortages and started promoting the need for national self-sufficiency. Both reactions highlight how in the case of international trade, the pandemic set national interests at odds with one another.

From an efficiency perspective, ambitions to be self-sufficient can come at a steep cost, which in the current circumstances can have serious public health consequences. When hockey equipment maker Bauer started producing plastic face shields in Canada for six dollars apiece, this was about five times as expensive as the same product made in China. One way to avoid such inefficiencies is to have enforceable country commitments to avoid export restraints of essential goods during crises, but this may not be politically palatable in every country. Another approach would be to defuse fears of shortages, to prevent a "run on export restrictions." To achieve this, one strategy would be to limit the market concentration of essential goods, to ensure that a single country does not produce a majority of the world's vaccines, as is now the case. The multilateral trade regime could, for instance, make room for temporary trade restrictions to allow states to protect certain producers and thus ensure less concentration in essential industries.

Another defining feature of the emergency phase is the opening of the *fiscal* floodgates, at least in countries that have the capacity to do so. Most countries affected by COVID-19 launched record stimulus packages. The size of the U.S. fiscal stimulus package represented almost 15 percent of the country's gross domestic product (GDP) (IMF 2021). However, this policy convergence occurred due to a lack of clear alternatives rather than as a coordinated global crisis response. Initially, most countries' responses included some form of unemployment benefit, tax rebates, and food support for the vulnerable. As expected, we are seeing more divergence in COVID-related policies as countries have entered the recovery phase. As more policy options become available, the political preferences of different governments have started to manifest themselves.

In the short term, the fiscal stimulus helped to cushion the unequal impact of the crisis on different population groups. Vulnerable populations are not only more likely to contract the virus, but they are also more likely to lose their jobs and find themselves unable to face the resulting economic hardship without assistance. For example, the Black population of Chicago represents just under a third of the general population but made up more than 70 percent of COVID-related deaths (Alobuia et al. 2020). Generally speaking, therefore, fiscal stimulus is amply justified. However, these expenses will have knock-on effects in the future, notably by putting pressure on public budgets.

Obviously, this budgetary pressure will weigh even more heavily on governments in the developing world, where resources are already scarce. In our view, as in the view of our colleagues who wrote the developing world chapter, *rich countries should provide more financial assistance to developing countries, in order to support their public health responses and mitigate economic hardships over the medium and long terms*. G20 countries agreed to suspend debt payments of $12 billion from poor country debtors between June 2020 and June 2021, but this is unlikely to be sufficient. Analyses of funds made available to poor countries in response to the crises show a limited increase in outright development assistance—including for instance an additional $7 billion coming from the Development Assistance Committee (DAC)—while the bulk of extra funding has come through loans such as those of the World Bank Group (OECD 2021, section 9). Compared to the estimated $16 trillion of economic stimulus in 2020, current efforts in development aid have to be considered less than a drop in the bucket. The pandemic sparked a global economic crisis, and it should be met with a coordinated foreign aid response.

In terms of *monetary policy*, central bankers around the world reacted to COVID-19 by reverting to the play book developed during the 2008 financial crisis: they launched a new round of asset purchases (quantitative easing) by which central banks buy securities from the financial sector and thus inject liquidity into the economy. Central bankers used this unconventional policy instrument because their more conventional tool, the interest rate, was already near 0 percent, which did not give them much room to manoeuvre.

Capital market liquidity shortages in mid-March 2020 suggested that central bank intervention was indeed appropriate. However, the scale of the intervention was surprising: between mid-March and mid-May 2020, the U.S. Federal Reserve alone expanded its balance sheet by $3 trillion through the acquisition of financial assets. By comparison, from July–December 2008 its balance sheet grew by "only"

$1 trillion (Board of Governors of the Federal Reserve System, n.d.). Several experts expressed concern that this radical response defied the monetary policy maxim requiring central banks to favour a more measured initial crisis response. In addition, this giant liquidity injection is likely to have significant unintended consequences that we discuss in more detail below.

Globally, the coordinated monetary policy response led by the U.S. Federal Reserve stands in contrast to the more nationalist and protectionist impulses in trade. The Federal Reserve provided unprecedented access to U.S. dollars, the main global reserve currency, by extending massive swap lines to other central banks worldwide. The value of these swap and credit lines jumped from $45 million in early March 2020 to $397 billion on 9 April 2020 (Collins, Potter, and Truman 2020, 54). For the first time, the Fed also provided money to foreign central banks via a mechanism akin to quantitative easing, by buying their Treasury bills. These measures aimed to prevent an appreciation of the U.S. dollar, which would have put pressure on those with dollar-denominated debt and potentially triggered an outflow of "hot money" from developing countries.

In sum, we can classify the international policy responses of the emergency phase into two categories. First, there were *policies arising from the clash of national interests*, such as export restrictions. Second, there were *policies that reflect a temporary alignment of interests*, such as the adoption of similar fiscal stimuli or the actions of the Fed. While the latter represents a form of U.S. leadership, this is a one-way response intended primarily to prevent markets key to U.S. interests from collapsing rather than an intervention motivated to serve the global good.

What we have not seen is a *cooperative* international economic response to the COVID-19 crisis. The defining feature of cooperation is that governments accept constraints on their behaviour or financial commitments that may not be in their narrowly defined, short-term self-interest. For instance, we did not see a global compact on how to allocate personal and medical protective equipment, but instead witnessed wild and competitive bidding for these vital resources. This lack of cooperation is in stark difference to the emergency period of the Great Recession of 2008 when G20 countries coordinated a large fiscal stimulus and committed to resist protectionist trade measures. In the recovery and aftermath phases, an effective response to the pandemic and its economic fallout will require genuine cooperation.

The danger, especially in a political climate already prone to populism, lies in the temptation for governments to favour non-cooperative behaviour that will yield collectively suboptimal results.

The Recovery Phase

How should public policy promote economic recovery in the wake of COVID-19? Against the background of developments in the emergency phase and based on experience from previous crises, there are a number of foreseeable pressure points and potential responses.

Starting once again with *trade*, the immediate focus on self-reliance in essential goods is likely to give way to more typical mercantilist policies that call for import restrictions and export promotion. When businesses are struggling for financial survival, governments are tempted to support local firms by shielding them from foreign competition with import tariffs and export subsidies. In the wake of the Great Recession of 2008, the trade regime successfully withstood such pressures. But countries' commitment to multilateral rules has considerably weakened in the interim, with the United States pulling out of the Trans-Pacific Partnership and threatening to pull out of the North American Free Trade Agreement (NAFTA, which, as of 1 July 2020, became known as the Canada-United States-Mexico Free Trade Agreement). Yet it is the United States' blocking appointments of new members to the Appellate Body of the World Trade Organization (WTO) since 2019 that may be most worrisome in this respect. It is through its dispute settlement mechanism that the WTO has been most effective in maintaining cooperation over the last two decades. With the current deadlock over judicial appointments, rulings may not be adopted once they are appealed, and may thus lack legal force. The result may be growing impunity, and protectionism on a level not seen for decades.

Initial debates about the dangers of global value chains have added fuel to the fire, giving a nationalist twist to mercantilist policies. Calling offshoring "a lemming-like desire for efficiency," U.S. trade representative Robert Lighthizer (2020) called for the dismantling of global value chains to "bring the jobs back to America." Japan has similarly promised subsidies to Japanese companies that are willing to bring production back to Japan from China. Global leaders need to embrace a renewed commitment to multilateralism in order to prevent a protectionist spiral. But without U.S. leadership, and with growing fissures between China and the United States, such international trade cooperation may not be possible. On the contrary, if anything the current trend points in the opposite direction, as evident for instance from the debate in Europe on how to resist "economic coercion" by bolstering economic sovereignty through measures ranging from a European export bank to a stronger role for the Euro in international currency markets.

Turning to *fiscal policy*, the second stage of the 2008 financial crisis provides a valuable lesson for public finances during the recovery phase. The 2008 U.S. subprime mortgage crisis and its global shockwaves were followed by a sovereign debt crisis in Europe in 2010–2012. With debt-to-GDP ratios soaring after the subprime crisis, many countries came under pressure from international financial markets. Several Eurozone members unable to use independent monetary policies to adjust were hit especially hard. Many countries reacted to this pressure with fiscal austerity—that is, they cut back government spending to rebalance their books. This strategy was a disaster and widely condemned as a result (e.g., Blyth 2013). Cutting social assistance, health, and education especially disadvantaged the most vulnerable members of society, who in many cases had already suffered disproportionate economic hardship during the crisis.

How can a similar scenario be avoided after COVID-19? There is no one-size-fits-all solution, but here are two general recommendations. First, fiscal policy during recovery should focus on spending and on bringing economies back to the pre-crisis growth trend. International organizations such as the G20, the International Monetary Fund (IMF) and the Organisation for Economic Co-operation and Development (OECD) need to work toward a *coordinated* stimulus effort. Coordination in the form of spending targets is important in part because one or two major countries breaking ranks and pursuing a lower taxation *cum* austerity strategy risk undermining the collective effort. The coordination should extend to developing countries, whose budget constraints will make sustained recovery spending difficult to impossible. Second, as we shall discuss below, finance ministries across the globe will have to cooperate to tap into additional sources of revenue.

In the context of *monetary policy*, central bankers and those responsible for setting their mandates must take several concerns into account. On the one hand, they will have to keep an eye on inflation which, for the first time in years, has been exceeding policy targets in many countries since 2021. We now know that this increase represents more than a temporary blip reflecting the rebound from low prices in 2020 as well as supply chain bottlenecks, but instead amounts to a more permanent policy challenge. On the other hand, especially in light of the more and more powerful policy tools they employ, central banks need to become more sensitive to concerns that reach beyond classic price stability objectives.

First, monetary policy has become less and less effective in recent years. One problem is that central banks have to rely on the financial sector to implement monetary policy. When they inject liquidity into the economy, they do not control where this liquidity ends up. Instead of translating into real economic activity, it increasingly accrues in asset markets such as real estate or stock markets. As a result, central banks must inject "excess" liquidity into the economy in order to produce a given impact on the rate of inflation. *In the future, meeting inflation and employment mandates could require them to adopt policies that bypass the private financial sector.*

Second, and as a direct consequence of this broken monetary policy transmission mechanism, the large liquidity injections characteristic of unconventional monetary policy can significantly increase wealth inequalities (De Haan and Eijffinger 2016; White 2012). When central banks conduct asset purchases, they tend to have little control over how the liquidity injected into the economy is used. When liquidity injections drive up asset markets rather than stimulating real economic activity, they disproportionately benefit wealthy asset holders. Without counterbalancing interventions, the staggering liquidity injections in the wake of COVID-19 is exacerbating the trend towards rising wealth inequality. In fact, a look at stock market indices suggests that we are already witnessing these consequences, with stocks handily beating their pre-COVID levels while the real economy languishes in the doldrums.

Third, the Fed's creation of swap lines for other central banks during the COVID-19 emergency presented it with a policy dilemma. Sticking to its mandate required the Fed to roll back these international liquidity measures as soon as financial stability permitted, whereas maintaining swap lines in the medium term promised to help international trade recover. The Fed chose the first route and revoked the swap lines in December 2021, but the dilemma points to a more fundamental issue: while opening swap lines during the COVID-19 emergency was certainly welcome and in stark contrast to other protectionist trends in U.S. policy, it also reflects persistent global dependence on the U.S. dollar and on the Federal Reserve, a dependence which contributes to cross-national economic vulnerabilities and antagonisms (Committee on the Global Financial System 2020).

Finally, another lesson from the 2008 global financial crisis lies in the link between fiscal and monetary policy. Some observers have suggested that fiscal austerity post-2008 would not have been possible without the expansionary monetary policy pursued by central banks.[1] In other words, without the cover provided by central banks, many governments would have been under pressure to provide more fiscal stimulus and not to cut government programs. On their own, unconventional monetary policies and austerity measures each increase inequalities, but the combination is self-reinforcing and devastating. In the COVID-19 recovery phase, countries would do well to avoid this combination. Monetary policy has stabilized financial markets for the moment, but long-term recovery requires sustained fiscal intervention.

The Aftermath

The pandemic has further exposed structural weaknesses in our current global institutions. For the second time in just over a decade, a crisis has laid bare the real social, political, and economic vulnerabilities of a global economic system with high specialization and market interconnectedness. Such globalization served as a potent vehicle for financial crisis contagion during the Great Recession of 2008–2009 and then for literal viral contagion during the COVID-19 pandemic. These twin crises have progressively weakened the trade regime and have boosted nationalist tendencies that reinforce fears of the Other. While the problems are by no means new, the pandemic has added a sense of urgency to addressing them and, at least temporarily, has opened a window of opportunity for reform. Importantly, fundamental reforms do not have to wait until the recovery phase is over. Indeed, they might be more politically feasible with the crisis fresh in our minds. Instead, what distinguishes the aftermath phase is the opportunity to deal with underlying structural issues that, if addressed successfully, would reduce the detrimental impact of future crises.

We are always gearing up to fight the last crisis, and this time will be no exception: it is likely that in the wake of COVID-19 countries will allocate significant resources to public health preparedness and cooperation. However, the next crisis will just as likely come from another corner. A series of climate-change-induced shocks to agricultural production, a Chinese economic collapse due to unsustainable debt, a real-estate bubble in OECD countries—the possible triggers are many, but they will all test the same economic institutions and practices. States will face growing incentives to favour domestic producers at the expense of foreign producers. Individual governments will seek to capture more tax revenue from multinationals in ways that might make an effective global tax regime less likely to emerge. Central banks will need to act if elected officials hesitate, but they may lack the means to do so. Governments have a common interest in developing effective medical responses to COVID-19. By contrast, the pandemic's economic fallout can lead to clashing short-term interests, with detrimental long-term implications. It is thus in the economic sphere that the need for institutional change to facilitate genuine global cooperation is greatest. How might we achieve it?

Looking to *trade*, one lesson of the global recession triggered by the financial crisis in 2008 is that domestic imbalances have a way of spilling over internationally. Regions hardest hit by trade competition are more likely to harbour anti-immigrant attitudes, vote for nationalist leaders, and demand trade protection. Trade adjustment policies that compensate those most exposed to import competition can significantly dampen these negative effects: regions in the United States with greater trade adjustment measures for workers in exposed industries were less likely to support protectionist measures (Kim and Pelc 2021). If the steel worker in Michigan or the farmer in the Midwest does not feel left behind, they are less likely to fall for populist slogans. In other words, *by confronting domestic imbalances, states can do much to relieve stress on the global system.* Such redistribution policies are politically fraught in many countries, but a system of global trade that does not manage to achieve a more equitable distribution of the gains from trade will always be subject to instability.

International cooperation in trade is far more extensive than in fiscal or monetary policy. As a consequence, it is also the arena in which the international community stands to lose the most if current institutions and practices break down under the pressure of a crisis such as COVID-19. Can the G20 commit to controlling a wave of protectionism? Can the WTO avert a crisis of legitimacy similar to that currently experienced by the World Health Organization (WHO)? These remain open questions. The answers will depend on the ability of the international community, and in particular the world's two largest economies, the United States and China, to re-create a climate that is more conducive to international cooperation than national competition. An early test of this will be whether the United States and the European Union are able to resolve the current impasse over the dispute settlement mechanism at the WTO, which has centred on its Appellate Body. Without an authoritative means of interpreting global trade rules, members are unlikely to respect either the letter or the spirit of the law. A number of initiatives have emerged among WTO members to try and push through reform in hopes of maintaining cooperation during the global recovery. The Ottawa Group, made up of 14 countries, is among these, and it has offered a number of proposals since the start of the pandemic. Tellingly, neither the United States nor China are part of the group. There is also a growing consensus that countries need to be given the policy space to strike a balance between economic independence and integration and manage supply chain vulnerabilities without generating excessive redundancies and inefficiencies. Yet a successful global project around which the international community can rally may prove decisive.

As to *fiscal policy*, where will governments find the revenue necessary to plug the enormous hole that COVID-19 will have torn into their finances? For many developing countries with a narrow tax base, raising sufficient revenue to cover the shortfalls caused by the pandemic will simply be impossible without significant change to century-old norms. The current G20 agreement to temporarily suspend debt servicing for low-income countries will not be enough (Berglöf, Brown, and Farrar 2020). The international community should put in place arrangements to *forgive developing-country debt*, and dollar-denominated debt in particular, which has accrued due to COVID-19-related spending.

Even for richer countries, raising more revenue is not a straightforward exercise. Take the example of Italy and its €2.4 trillion pre-COVID national debt—130 percent of GDP and rising. The main reason that investors have not started asking for higher risk premia for holding Italian debt is that the European Central Bank (ECB) could not afford an Italian sovereign debt default and is providing a credible backstop. This is hardly a sustainable solution. Italy and other countries in a similar situation could raise indirect taxes such as a value-added tax (VAT), but unless carefully designed, such taxes can be regressive. Just like austerity policies, they disproportionately burden the poor who spend a higher percentage of their income on consumption.

A more promising alternative is to identify revenue sources that make the *tax system more progressive*, thus easing the inegalitarian impact of the pandemic. This leaves two options: higher marginal tax rates for the wealthy and higher tax rates on capital income (corporate profits, dividends, capital gains). The former can be done unilaterally. Although skeptics argue that this will reduce high earners' incentives to work, several studies suggest that the labour supply of high earners is relatively insensitive to income tax rates (Saez, Slemrod, and Giertz 2012). Moreover, social emergencies such as pandemics or wars historically boost solidarity and thus open a window of opportunity for governments to ask their wealthiest citizens to contribute more.

By contrast, taxing capital is more challenging and requires international cooperation in the face of international capital mobility and tax competition. Since the launch of its "harmful tax competition" campaign at the end of the 1990s, the OECD has made significant progress, especially in curtailing individual tax evasion. Addressing corporate tax avoidance has proved significantly more difficult, notably because the interests of different countries do not necessarily align. The fiscal bottlenecks that the COVID-19 crisis will create might be the catalyst needed for effective reform in this domain.

The OECD Inclusive Framework has recently developed a two-pronged proposal for *international tax reform* (World Economic Forum 2019). The first pillar aims to respond to the changing nature of business models in the digital age by allowing countries to tax corporations "with sustained and significant involvement" in their economies even if the corporations do not have a physical presence there. The second pillar, already adopted in the fall of 2021, introduces a global minimum corporate tax rate of 15 percent, which reduces the benefit of profit shifting as a corporate tax avoidance strategy. The challenge moving forward lies in ensuring that the effectiveness of this new tool does not get diminished through exemptions and loopholes.

For much of the 1990s and early 2000s, *monetary policy* was widely considered to be a technocratic exercise that would not interfere significantly with other policy objectives. This changed with the global financial crisis and the introduction of unconventional monetary policy. Most now understand that central bank actions have significant unintended consequences in realms ranging from economic inequality to climate change. The era of central bank independence with its narrow focus on price stability is coming to an end, as demonstrated by the Fed's softening of their inflation target in August 2020, and despite the recent uptick in inflation rates. If central banks want to retain their operational autonomy, the new paradigm will have to take the unintended consequences of monetary policy into account.

Two interrelated reforms can address this new reality. First, central banks need to repair the transmission mechanisms of monetary policy. In other words, they need to make sure that their policy instruments actually have the intended effects on price stability and financial stability. On the one hand, they should ramp up the *conditionality requirements of their asset purchases*. Concretely, a financial institution should only benefit from an asset purchase program if it channels the resulting liquidity to the real economy. On the other hand, central bankers should *experiment with policies such as helicopter money* (direct monetary disbursements to the public) that bypass the financial system altogether and thus promise to be more effective. Neither of these reforms are likely to see the light of day if pursued unilaterally. Instead, the central banks of the largest economies should cooperate to move ahead with these reforms in synchronized fashion, thus creating incentives for others to follow.

Second, governments should expand central bank mandates to give central bankers the power to combat counterproductive side effects such as exacerbating economic inequality, especially where governments themselves are unable or reluctant to address them directly. What should the ideal mandate of a central bank be under these circumstances? As leading monetary theorists acknowledge (Rogoff 1985), those in charge of pursuing price and financial stability should take costly side effects into account. Changing central bank mandates *to make monetary policy sensitive to distributional concerns* represents one possible path for reform (Dietsch, Claveau, and Fontan 2018). To take the concrete example of COVID-19 measures, it is clear that injecting trillions of dollars into the world economy through current means will deepen economic inequalities both within and across countries. With expanded mandates, central bankers could explore alternative, less inegalitarian ways to achieve the same results, as well as increase coordination with fiscal authorities so that their policies complement rather than clash with one another. Helicopter money or asset purchases geared toward promoting a green economy are two examples of monetary policies likely to be better aligned with broader policy objectives. While the European Central Bank and the Bank of England have already taken significant steps in the direction of including concerns of inequality and of climate change in their decision-making, in the Canadian context, the renewal of the Bank of Canada's mandate in 2021 extended the status quo and there are no signs for this conservative approach to change in the foreseeable future.

Conclusion

Almost four years on, it is clear that the COVID-19 crisis has put significant strain on international institutions. In particular, it has exacerbated national and global inequalities. Thus far, governments have not taken sufficient concrete measures to contain these inequalities in some of the ways we have described. A more cooperatively minded Biden administration in Washington has made a difference, but not to the extent hoped for and anticipated by some. The only effective way to contain the impact of COVID-19 on the international economy is through *genuine global cooperation*.

Note

1.   The direction of causality between fiscal and monetary policy is not entirely clear. Did loose monetary policy render austerity possible, or did austerity make loose monetary policy necessary? Either way, the combination of the two is undesirable (Green and Lavery 2015).

References

Alobuia, Wilson M., Nathan P. Dalva-Baird, Joseph D. Forrester, Eran Bendavid, Jay Bhattacharya, and Electron Kebebew. 2020. "Racial Disparities in Knowledge, Attitudes and Practices Related to Covid-19 in the USA." *Journal of Public Health* 42, no. 3 (September): 470–478.

Berglöf, Erik, Gordon Brown, and Jeremy Farrar. 2020. "Letter to Governments of the G20 Nations." *VoxEU CEPR*, April 7, 2020. https://voxeu.org/article/letter-governments-g20-nations.

Blyth, Mark. 2013. *Austerity – The History of a Dangerous Idea*. Oxford: Oxford University Press.

Board of Governors of the Federal Reserve System. n.d. "Credit and Liquidity Programs and the Balance Sheet. Recent Balance Sheet Trends." Accessed on March 12, 2021. https://www.federalreserve.gov/monetarypolicy/bst_recenttrends.htm.

Collins, Christopher G., Simon M. Potter, and Edwin M. Truman. 2020. "Enhancing Central Bank Cooperation in the Covid-19 Pandemic."

In *PIIE Briefing 20-1: How the G20 Can Hasten Recovery from Covid-19*, edited by Maurice Obstfeld and Adam S. Posen, 52–56. Washington, D.C.: Peterson Institute for International Economics Briefing. https://www.piie.com/publications/piie-briefings/how-g20-can-hasten-recovery-covid-19.

Committee on the Global Financial System. 2020. "US Dollar Funding: An International Perspective." Bank of International Settlements CGFS Papers no. 65. https://www.bis.org/publ/cgfs65.pdf.

De Haan, Jakob, and Sylvester Eijffinger. 2016. "The Politics of Central Bank Independence." Dutch National Bank Working Paper no. 539. https://papers.ssrn.com/sol3/papers.cfm?abstract_id=2887931.

Dietsch, Peter, François Claveau, and Clément Fontan. 2018. *Do Central Banks Serve the People?* Cambridge: Polity Press.

Green, Jeremy, and Scott Lavery. 2015. "The Regressive Recovery: Distribution, Inequality and State Power in Britain's Post-Crisis Political Economy." *New Political Economy* 20 (6): 894–923.

IMF (International Monetary Fund). 2021. "Policy Responses to COVID-19 – United States of America." Last modified January 7, 2021. https://www.imf.org/en/Topics/imf-and-covid19/Policy-Responses-to-COVID-19#U

Kim, Sung Eun, and Krzysztof Pelc. 2021. "The Politics of Trade Adjustment vs. Trade Protection." *Comparative Political Studies* 54 (13): 2354–2381.

Lighthizer, Robert E. 2020. "The Era of Offshoring U.S. Jobs Is Over." *The New York Times*, May 11, 2020. https://www.nytimes.com/2020/05/11/opinion/coronavirus-jobs-offshoring.html.

OECD (Organisation for Co-operation and Development). 2020. *Development Co-operation Report 2020: Learning from Crises, Building Resilience.* Paris: OECD Publishing. https://doi.org/10.1787/f6d42aa5-en.

Rogoff, Kenneth. 1985. "The Optimal Degree of Commitment to an Intermediate Monetary Target." *Quarterly Journal of Economics* 100, no. 4 (November): 1169–1189.

Saez, Emannuel, Joel Slemrod, and Seth H. Giertz. 2012. "The Elasticity of Taxable Income with Respect to Marginal Income Tax Rates: A Critical Review." *Journal of Economic Literature* 50, no. 1 (March): 3–50.

White, William R. 2012. "Ultra Easy Monetary Policy and the Law of Unintended Consequences." Federal Reserve Bank of Dallas Globalization and Monetary Policy Institute Working Paper no. 126. https://www.dallasfed.org/~/media/documents/institute/wpapers/2012/0126.pdf.

World Economic Forum. 2019. "Corporate Tax, Digitalization and Globalization." White Paper, December 2019. http://www3.weforum.org/docs/WEF_Corporate_Tax_Digitalization_and_Globalization.pdf.

CHAPTER 4

Information Technology

Karim Benyekhlef, Anthony Amicelle,
Nicholas King, and Samuel Tanner

The pandemic highlighted—if proof were even needed—advanced societies' growing dependence on digital infrastructure. Networking—which has been going on since the emergence of the consumer internet in the mid-1990s—and the digitization of human activities since the 1970s are major trends that the COVID-19 health crisis has accelerated. Businesses shuttering, millions of workers losing their jobs, and the near-complete shutdown of all economic activity caused an economic crisis, which the use of digital technology then helped to mitigate, in particular through telework and online shopping and services. Governments were able to continue operating, as were companies in the tertiary sector (services), thereby cushioning the blow and avoiding more devastating societal disruption.

This situation has certainly boosted the stock market value of the major internet operators. However, beyond the naïve celebration of a digital society, digital platform-specific problems—already identified pre-pandemic—remain. If anything, they have gotten worse. Crises inevitably give rise to rumours, malicious gossip, lies, discriminatory and defamatory comments, and fake news. These sad realities are serious threats to countries' political stability. They undermine the trust that lies at the heart of the democratic functioning of our societies and threaten social harmony. The COVID-19 crisis also highlighted the inequalities in access to technology. For example, when it comes to teleworking or having access to public services, those who live in remote areas and do not benefit from the technological facilities available in urban environments may be at a disadvantage.

However, crises often have one thing in common—they weaken individual rights and freedoms in the name of a sacred unity against evil. Debates over tracking applications designed to limit and prevent the spread of COVID-19 illustrate the delicate trade-offs that decision-makers must make when managing a crisis. In this case, the right to personal data protection—a subset of the right to privacy—and the imperatives of public health are in conflict. Close monitoring of individual behaviour would make it possible to better manage health risks. Nowadays, it goes without saying that this kind of monitoring involves digital technology (i.e., the increasingly precise and invasive monitoring of our digital interactions). This is a broad and complex issue, as it involves the belief—often akin to magical thinking—that technology is the only adequate response to collective problems (i.e., so-called "techno-solutionism") (Morozov 2014). This belief existed before the pandemic.

In this chapter, we will address two issues: (1) the regulation of platforms, which are the main drivers of the digital lives of the vast majority of citizens and public and private administrations; and (2) the surveillance of individuals through an increased use of these platforms in our socioeconomic interactions—personal, civic, and professional. Platform regulation raises the issue of controlling the content shared on them and the monitoring of individuals raises questions about how to protect personal data.

Infodemic Reigns

Contemporary societies suffer from information overload, which leads to significant risks of both misinformation and disinformation. In a pandemic context, the term "infodemic" is aptly used to describe the viral spread of false information, particularly about the pandemic itself and its possible solutions. Therefore, it is crucial for citizen engagement, security, and social regulation to be able to verify and determine the accuracy of the content to which we are exposed.

The notion of an infodemic is more broadly linked to the phenomenon of "fake news"—false information deliberately developed and disseminated in traditional media, but primarily on digital platforms, to confuse and influence social debate, thereby sowing doubt. Fake news can also take the form of "deep fakes"—audiovisual manipulations powered by artificial intelligence and deep learning that use simulation to generate words or actions and attribute them to people who have never said or done them.

Fake news creates a crisis of confidence among citizens, the media, and public, private, and political institutions. It also causes destabilization and tension between social, ethnic, and political groups and fuels community bias and discrimination. In the political and social context of heightening racial tensions and the questioning of policing practices and the role of the police—highlighted in spring 2020 by the Black Lives Matter movement—search engines, including Google, share some of the responsibility for the rise in racial discrimination. Safiya Umoja Noble (2018) showed the extent to which Google search results related to Black Lives Matter linked to infamous conspiracy sites, analyzing the information creep and heavy impacts it has on groups that are subject to discrimination.

Whether it stems from manipulative discourse, deep fakes, or technological bias, fake news is a source of truncated, inaccurate, biased, prejudicial, and discriminatory representations. It could influence people's social construction processes while giving shape to alternative realities that affect beliefs and blur the boundaries between truth, misinformation, and lies.

Beyond fake news and propaganda, the COVID-19 pandemic drew our attention to another troubling aspect of the information ecosystem: the role of expertise, particularly scientific expertise. Typically, the production of scientific knowledge and its influence on policy making are long-term processes that occur away from the public eye. However, the role of scientific experts, particularly epidemiologists and infectious disease modellers, was unusually visible during the pandemic. For example, models of COVID-19 impacts produced by experts at Imperial College, Harvard University, and the Institute for Health Metrics and Evaluation were widely shared on social networks and were cited by politicians in the United Kingdom, the United States, and elsewhere as having crucially influenced decision-making. However, as with other types of information, these models were met with a swift and vehement reaction, as the scientists' work was repeatedly criticized on social media and misrepresented by the very politicians who had initially referenced it approvingly. The pandemic illustrated—and perhaps accelerated—the long-standing phenomenon of populist leaders using platforms where information of uneven quality circulates to attack scientific expertise and judgment and the privileged position experts have long held publicly.

New Relationships with the Truth

Disinformation—the most popular forms of which are propaganda and conspiracy theories—is not new. However, the capacity of the contemporary media ecosystem, including digital platforms, has made it a powerful vector of public amplification, dissemination, and virality. These platforms consist of a set of applications and software based on an ideology known as surveillance capitalism (Zuboff 2019). The technological architecture of Web 2.0 allows for user-generated content to be created and shared, but it also interferes with users' choices regarding how they organize their lives and relate to (or read) their environment (Van Dijck 2013). Technological communication capabilities (including artificial intelligence, big data, algorithms, and digital platforms) and their biases profoundly influence the information economy, exponentially boosting information dissemination and penetration capabilities and enabling the advent of what some call "computational propaganda" (DiResta 2018).

This increase in fake news is happening at a time when our relationship with the truth has transformed. Some believe we are in a so-called "post-truth" era, established no longer on verified facts, but instead on emotions, beliefs, and feelings (McIntyre 2018). In other words, public opinion is less influenced by objective facts than by the appeal of emotions and personal beliefs. This phenomenon is not unique to our contemporary context; Robert K. Merton asserted as far back as the 1940s that "public definitions of a situation (prophecies or predictions) become an integral part of the situation and thus affect subsequent developments. This is peculiar to human affairs. It is not found in the world of nature" (Merton 2016, 506). Contrary to the Orwellian prophecy of *1984*, which imagined a ministry imposing the Truth on all individuals, in today's media ecosystem everyone can share it straight from their keyboard with minimal technological expertise. This capacity for amplification and virality makes it possible to launder one's vile notions (fake news) through the public information economy, to potentially detrimental effects.

Regulating Platforms to Control the Flow of Information

The major platforms (e.g., Facebook, X, Amazon, and Google) have centralized the internet.[1] Although the original internet was based on a completely decentralized architecture that facilitated anonymous browsing with no content control, business requirements have imposed an additional layer of personal identification and content control to ensure transactions are secure. Business demands a safe and secure transactional environment and — consequently — the development of control measures and the imposition of constraints. This centralization has conferred considerable — if not excessive — power on the major platforms, as the platform operator's control derives directly from the technical architecture in question and the internal rules of use. It is interesting to note that, in this context, the global aspect of the internet is no longer an impediment to the normative action of the state, which can institute a variety of standards to govern cyberspace activities.

In the early days of the internet, prescriptive government intervention was ruled out in favour of self-regulation so that operators could develop viable business models. This notion that actors should be left to conduct their own business is reflected in the immunity from prosecution platforms that content hosts are granted for the content they house, similar to the model used in the days of common carriers (e.g., Bell Canada), which could not be held liable for the content of telephone conversations on their networks. In 1996, the United States adopted section 230 of the Communications Decency Act, under which platforms cannot be held responsible for content posted on their networks. This absolute — or near absolute — immunity grants them privileged status, as — unlike newspaper publishers — they are not required to filter and control the content that is broadcast or published. This is a major advantage that was granted at a time in the internet's history when business models had not yet been established and no one knew how to monetize the web and how people used it.

In the wake of the pandemic, but also of the Black Lives Matter movement and the U.S. elections, social networks such as X, Facebook, Reddit, YouTube, and Twitch toughened their policies on false-information sharing (e.g., by issuing warnings or banning racist or hateful comments). Following the 6 January 2021 assault on the Capitol, former president Trump's X and Facebook accounts were permanently suspended because of the incitements to violence they contained. This raises the broader question of the status of these platforms (host or publisher?) and the sources of regulation because, while platforms now have codes of conduct and quasi-jurisdictional internal mechanisms, their self-regulation—perhaps even their immunity—is a major reason why so-called "putrid content," to which everyone on the major platforms has access, is proliferating (e.g., fake news, conspiracy theories, and defamatory, discriminatory, racist, and anti-Semitic content). Under U.S. law, platforms cannot be held liable for such content, and they are not even required to remove it once its criminal nature has been legally established. However, the major platforms are—first and foremost—subject to U.S. law. A form of extraterritoriality of U.S. law makes it more difficult to regulate platforms, although not impossible, as demonstrated by the European Union (EU) with the General Data Protection Regulation (GDPR), which also regulates the cross-border flow of European residents' personal data.

The pandemic did not change existing trends—those relating to fake news and those proposing to limit platforms' immunity or dismantle them. The centralization of the internet and major platforms' increased role mean that regulation is possible, even if it involves legal and—above all—political challenges. The dominance of U.S. platforms makes the U.S. government highly critical of any prescriptive action aimed at them. In the wake of an undoubtedly excessive interpretation of trade treaties, prescriptive actions appear suspicious at first glance, even though they may be perfectly legitimate. Take, for example, the regulation of personal data protection. A country has the right to ensure the protection of its citizens' privacy, without this being a non-tariff barrier to trade, which is prohibited by the rules of free trade.

To explain the upsurge in fake news, we also need to take a brief look at the disinformation shared on our platforms, often at the instigation of authoritarian countries. Disinformation is not a purely national phenomenon. Controlling information on digital platforms has become even more difficult because the internet has become an instrument of propaganda, manipulation, and cyberattacks. Russia is a major player in this digital disruption. China is also involved, often adopting Russian techniques and tactics (Charon and Vilmer 2021). Russia mobilizes information technology (IT) in the form of hybrid warfare, combining military and non-military activities, and employing non-state actors to take harmful action. In our case, these are obviously cyber actions often deployed by activists who are not officially attached to a state, but who act on their behalf (Henrotin 2018), as is the case with Russian hackers. As a result, Russia—imitated by China and other authoritarian states—is waging a veritable psychological war on social networks to poison relationships between the political authorities and citizens of certain countries, exacerbate social tensions, and—more generally—sow discord. In this respect, a report by the Institut de recherche stratégique de l'École militaire (IRSEM) clearly explains how China is waging this war using psychology and public opinion (Charon and Vilmer 2021). These actions help further spread "putrid content" and false information around the world according to the strategic objectives of the states behind them. These forms of interference are certainly an argument in favour of transforming these platforms into a public service, which would help curb these aggressive tactics by ensuring better content control, primarily through independent monitoring bodies. More on this later.

Recently, certain platforms—X in particular—have attempted to better control misleading or racist content. If such content emanates from political figures, a warning can be displayed to inform users of the inaccurate or otherwise misleading nature of the message. X recently did just this, urging users to confirm the veracity of published content in response to certain tweets by former president Donald Trump. However, platforms go even further when such vile content emanates from ordinary citizens or groups—they censor the posts or simply delete the accounts hosting them. The growing outrage we are seeing seemingly bolsters the claim that platforms do not want to act as judges of public discourse. Nevertheless, this new policy could be just temporary, destined to disappear in more favourable circumstances.

With the advent of vaccines and the introduction of "vaccine passports" to curb the COVID-19 pandemic, content questioning the quality or effectiveness of vaccines began to proliferate on social networks. For example, according to one anti-vaccine argument, RNA-messenger technology can alter one's genetic code and lead to more serious illnesses. Obviously, this false claim is based on a very poor understanding of this vaccine technology, but it can convince individuals not to get vaccinated, thus short-circuiting public vaccination campaigns. The risk of misinformation stems from an undoubtedly pernicious notion of freedom of expression, but it becomes majorly significant because of the lightning speed with which information is shared on platforms. This worrying public health situation calls for strict regulation of platform operators; regulation likely to better define the limits inherent in freedom of expression than the platforms' internal rules could. In addition, we know that platforms— through their algorithms—have the means to largely control not only how viral content goes and how widely it is shared, but also how it is shared. A report by the infodemic working group, under the Forum on Information and Democracy, recommends using legal rules to force these platforms to be more transparent. In particular, operators would be required to maintain an up-to-date document outlining the functions of their algorithms and how they affect the dissemination of information that is posted (Deloire et al. 2020). Platforms would also be required to disclose the amount of content their moderation teams or algorithms deem illegal, as well as why this content was deemed illegal (Deloire et al. 2020).

Reconciling Freedom of Expression and Information Monitoring

Therefore, it seems important to seize the opportunity this pandemic presents to take balanced platform regulation a step further. There are two suggestions that could accomplish this, thereby contributing to cleaner public discourse: (1) make some of these platforms public services, which would be subject to a specific regulatory body; and (2) give courts the power to judge the legality of content on the basis of immediate summary proceedings through a digital dispute-resolution platform (E-justice). Both suggestions are based on a fundamental premise—the importance of freedom of expression.[2]

In Canada, as in EU countries, freedom of expression is constitutionally protected, but it is not absolute. Certain types of speech have been—and still are—banned in our democratic spaces: defamation, hate speech, privacy breaches, and so forth.

However, in Canada, it is not illegal to share false news. In 1992, the Supreme Court of Canada's Zundel decision clearly stated that section 181 of the Criminal Code, which prohibits the spreading of false news, violated section 2(b) of the Canadian Charter of Rights and Freedoms, which guarantees freedom of expression.[3] The court acknowledged that a false statement can sometimes have a certain value and—above all—that it is difficult to determine conclusively whether it is completely false. Therefore, freedom of expression must be given priority in such cases. However, this declaration of unconstitutionality does not give *carte blanche* to every type of speech.

Other legal avenues, such as legislation on hate speech, defamation, trade secrets, or privacy breaches, ensure that public discourse is filtered. This is the legal context that prevailed pre-social media, and there is no reason to change course now that these platforms are the primary means of disseminating speech. In short, the various legislative instruments that govern public expression are sufficiently extensive to ensure responsible freedom of expression in our democratic societies.

Hate Content Regulation

Communication and discourse platforms like Facebook and X are now the preferred method of sharing information, in the broadest sense of the term. They have centralized the internet's communication capabilities, and it is difficult to deliver a message of any kind nowadays (e.g., political, commercial, social) without going through these channels. These platforms exercise a *de facto* monopoly on communication, which calls for a review of their practices and the appropriateness of maintaining them as they are, in the light of national competition policies. Pending such a review, it would be useful to consider them as a public communications service (like telephone companies) and — therefore — subjecting them to the oversight of a regulatory body, such as the Canadian Radio-television and Telecommunications Commission. The pandemic further underscored the general value of their operations, as, in many respects, they have helped foster social ties, maintain certain economic service activities and, more generally, uphold community life in a virtual setting.

From this perspective, there is a real possibility that these platforms could be deemed public services, which would enable greater government control over operators. For example, in addition to legislation, an oversight body could regulate both the economic conditions under which platforms operate and the conditions under which they are used. The foundations of such an oversight body can be found in the EU's Digital Services Act, which imposes obligations on platforms providing an online intermediary service. These obligations will be reinforced by a competent national authority and the creation of a European central body (Crichton 2021a). In the Digital Markets Act, the Commission acknowledges these platforms' power to control markets, conferring on them a new status — of "gatekeepers." As such, the control they exercise is subject to obligations and restrictions, but these obligations mainly concern competition law. This should be a first step toward designating these platforms as a public service.

The fact that the services these platforms offer are free of charge should not be an obstacle to such oversight, as it is well known that this gratuity is fictitious, given the commodification of users' personal data. The oversight body could thus ensure that platforms do editorial reviews of the content they host. However, this review is only possible if the platforms' existing immunity is modified in favour of a liability similar to that of newspaper publishers, which exercise control over the content they publish and face sanctions if it is illegal.

E-justice – An Additional Measure

Having a complementary measure in place would allow oversight bodies and platforms to avoid being both judge and party in the case of potentially unlawful content: this would involve allowing immediate referral to a judge who could rule on the content (interlocutory decision) within a very short timeframe and defer detailed examination to a later hearing, if necessary. Current technology makes it possible to resolve many disputes online, without the parties having to meet. The pandemic has boosted the use of IT in managing and processing legal cases, which has been reflected in the dematerialization of courtrooms, with some trials being held completely outside the walls of a courthouse, with all parties able to connect remotely using various videoconferencing tools. Legal proceedings are also being dematerialized through IT-based facilitatory measures (e.g., serving procedure documents using technology, e-filing and e-managing proceedings, and digitizing court files). Therefore, there is no reason why questions of lawfulness of content—in terms of freedom of expression and its recognized limits—should not be promptly submitted to a judge online. This is an effective response to the assertion that platforms cannot be the arbiters of freedom of expression.

The action of an oversight body, combined with treating platforms such as Facebook or X like public services and rapid online responses from a judge, should help resolutely mitigate the problems caused by fake news.

Protecting Individual Freedoms in Times of Crisis... and Beyond

The IT issues that came to light during the pandemic go far beyond platform regulation; they also include the challenge that government surveillance facilitated—even exacerbated—by technology, and often authorized by law, poses to both individual and collective freedoms.

Since the onset of the pandemic, many states have put systems in place that are commonly referred to as "health emergencies" (see also Chapter 8 on human rights). In short, these systems enable public authorities to impose the measures required to protect the health of the population. In Quebec, the declaration of a health emergency, its legal system, and how it is applied are set out in sections 118 et seq. of its Public Health Act. In France, this type of specific system had to be created, as it did not exist before the pandemic, though a general exception system did exist. We will leave it to others to question the relevance of creating such a system (see Beaud and Guérin-Bargues 2020). This new system was introduced when an emergency law to address the COVID-19 pandemic was adopted and entered into force.

Avoiding the Transposition of an Exceptional Legal System to an Ordinary One

All democratic states that dealt with the COVID-19 pandemic generally have similar provisions—or ones with similar effects. The measures implemented under such a state of emergency vary, ranging from organizing health services to imposing restrictions on individual and collective freedoms (bans on gatherings, potentially infringing on freedom of assembly and association, as well as the right to demonstrate; major restrictions on freedom of movement; the closure of services considered non-essential, which could be considered an infringement of freedom of enterprise) to limit the spread of a virus by reducing the risk of infection and—more generally—to protect the health of the population in the face of a serious health risk. As with any state of emergency, this means a shift from ordinary law to exceptional powers, which is one reason why declaring a state of emergency must be subject to strict oversight. In the cases of Quebec and France (which can be extrapolated easily to other countries with similar legal systems), there are specific rules for declaring a health emergency. In theory, the reasons for doing so, its duration, the procedures for extending it, and the mechanisms of checks and balances (through the executive, legislative, and judicial powers) must ensure the continuity of the democratic system and force a reverse switch from a state of exception to a state of ordinary law.

Given the infringements of freedoms that can be justified by a state of emergency, it is good that they are strictly regulated. However, caution must be exercised, as there are insidious ways in which measures that should never leave the framework of the state of emergency are brought into ordinary law. France has already shown that this is possible after having transposed certain oversight provisions into ordinary law in the wake of the attacks on 13 November 2015 (Champeil-Desplats 2017). The use of new technology that normalizes these infringements of rights and freedoms further increases this risk. With a view to balancing powers, we feel it is important to grant parliaments greater control over the way in which the executive exercises power in declaring and handling states of emergency.

Challenges and Uses of New Surveillance Technology

Some consider the pandemic to be the first case of global "policing," (i.e., enforcing rules through mechanisms of control and coercion, with a graduated set of measures for surveillance, health-risk management, and governance of associated forms of insecurity being implemented concomitantly in each state) (Sheptycki 2020). At this historic time of heightened social-control dynamics, the use of "new" technology has been examined with a critical eye, from police drones, thermal cameras, tools for modelling population movements using cell phone geolocation data, "or even [the] promotion of 'contact tracing' applications between individuals" (Tréguer 2020, 1). These applications have drawn the particular attention of both academics and the relevant national and international authorities, starting with the World Health Organization (WHO).

Fundamental rights-related problems have been at the heart of challenges to techno-solutionism, of which the promotion of tracking tools is just the latest example. These tools were touted as one of the preferred solutions for avoiding lockdowns and its impacts on freedom of movement and—by extension—on the economy. They have raised questions about both their effectiveness—particularly if their use is not coupled with a mass testing campaign—and their potential long-term impacts on the social acceptance of hitherto controversial public–private mobility monitoring devices (Bigo 2020). There have been widespread public calls in many countries to debate the relevance of these tools, to frame their purposes, and to create relative oversight mechanisms for their use. In this respect, the way contact tracing applications have been rolled out has differed from one country to another, some abandoning them altogether and others encouraging their use, usually on a voluntary basis.

However, the introduction of the vaccine passport in several liberal democracies has shown that restricting freedom of movement for public health reasons has not been subject to constitutional censure with regard to restrictions on access to places or activities deemed non-essential. Like the Quebec government, which imposed a vaccine passport from 2021 to 2022, the French Constitutional Council greenlit the introduction of a "health pass" (De Comarmont 2021), which would be mandatory even for non-emergency hospital appointments. "Experts" thus considered that the legal text was balanced and offered sufficient guarantees. Europe—more broadly—adopted the community health pass to enable travel between member states, and some countries have introduced a national health pass (Tobelem 2021). We can draw two conclusions from this information. First, in most of our liberal democracies, the courts consider restricting freedom of movement to be a proportionate and acceptable measure. Second, the public seems to accept this infringement of their freedoms, if polls on the acceptance of these measures[4] and vaccination rates—which have risen in several countries since they were announced—are to be believed.

As with policing and security issues in contemporary societies (the subject of several studies), the role new technologies play in pandemic management has by no means been forgotten. Important though they are, these technological developments and their use should not be overestimated, and the use of less high-tech—but no less pervasive—control and surveillance practices in the recent pandemic should not be overlooked.

In authoritarian countries such as China, the effectiveness of surveillance has more to do with the rapid mobilization of surveillance resources (particularly human resources). This mobilization—combined with strict measures imposed on the public and the economy of small- and medium-sized enterprises—has enabled effective surveillance. Digital tools, such as the Health Code, have been used to support already well-established surveillance.

The Logic of Whistleblowing in the Age of the Vigilant Society

The health emergency and the warlike rhetoric that accompanied it also led to a somewhat-unexpected resurgence of civic initiatives. One of these was controversial, as it stood in stark contrast to the general surge of generosity and solidarity—whistleblowing. A non-exhaustive survey of the international press carried out in April and May 2020 revealed how this phenomenon took hold in every corner of the world, from the middle-class neighbourhoods of northern Johannesburg, South Africa, to major Belgian and French cities, Canadian provinces, and New Zealand. Whether at the neighbourhood, municipal, regional, or national level, the situation was pretty much the same: there was an influx of calls—to the point of saturating emergency operations centres—about individuals suspected of violating lockdown rules. In Quebec, the scale of this phenomenon was measured by the public authorities' response: in an official video, provincial police representatives urged their fellow citizens "not to get paranoid."

On both sides of the Atlantic and the Pacific, this was all it took to rekindle the debate on whistleblowing as a (potential) civic act. People took different positions, from refusal in principle to civic duty, but they invariably stumbled over the definition of a clear dividing line between "good" reporting and "bad" tattling, with arguments generally centred on the seriousness of the acts deemed "health risks" and on the nature of individual motivations.

A video released by a Quebec police department[5] is based entirely on this distinction, with multiple examples and the following conclusion: "We must act in good faith, using judgment and common sense. We must not resort to extreme whistleblowing that clogs up our emergency call services." The message is unambiguous: "yes, we must blow the whistle," but we must do so "appropriately," and to do so, we must refer to the definitional criteria of "extenuating circumstances" provided by the state's repressive services. This phenomenon is by no means unique to Quebec (Rémy 2020; Kauffmann 2020); however, it varies from country to country depending on their sociohistorical relationship to the logics of citizen whistleblowing. In France, a departmental prefect issued an order aimed at requisitioning rule breakers to "prevent and report to the forces of law and order" any breaches of lockdown rules (Delouche-Bertolasi 2020). Following an outcry, the order was rescinded after only a few days. In

New Zealand, the online COVID-19 L4 breach form the police department created for the public remained accessible and was a victim of its own success.

The debate—here and elsewhere—no longer seems to be limited to the merits of whistleblowing in and of itself, but rather to the conditions under which it takes place. Are we witnessing the advent of a resurgence of suspicion and whistleblowing as instruments of the state and techniques of government?

Just as the use of new technologies has become commonplace, this apparent breakdown cannot be overestimated, as whistleblowing is already a standard tool of public action that goes well beyond the usual figures of the "crow," the informer, or the protected witness (Brodeur and Jobard 2005). Many public policies give space to the so-called citizen "informer," a term whose etymology refers precisely to denunciation, whether in the form of a call to a dedicated telephone line or a form to complete. While anti-terrorism policies are certainly the most striking illustration of this, they do not exhaust initiatives encouraging everyone to report suspicious behaviour, individuals, or things. In Quebec and Canada—as elsewhere—there are plenty of examples, from the tax and financial market authorities' "whistleblower programs," to the "web form for voluntarily reporting suspicions of money laundering" to the appropriate federal agency, or Canada Border Services Agency's "toll-free line" for "reporting suspicious activity at the border, a marriage of convenience," and so forth.

Therefore, the current debate on surveillance and social control in the era of health emergencies would benefit from being presented differently, in the light of a general trend toward enhancing these more or less high-tech political techniques, the definition and legitimate use of which state representatives want to continue to monopolize. In this respect, the origins, meaning, and contours of this vigilant society remain in question, as does its current evolution. Is this growing appeal to the citizen simply part of a wider process of transforming state response techniques, thereby encouraging everyone to assume responsibilities that were not or are no longer under their jurisdiction? In the age of social media and at a time of crisis that has led to unprecedented social anxiety, to what extent is it effective, worsened, or even overwhelmed and challenged by competing forms of vigilantism?

Similarly, while state use of digital surveillance tools has steadily increased during the pandemic, the high-tech industry's long-term role and increasingly pervasive effects within our societies are unknown. The new public–private partnerships in this field and the strong relationships between digital giants and governments the world over—from democratic to authoritarian regimes—are undoubtedly one of the most significant legacies of this pandemic. We now need to understand how, to what extent, and with what implications these recent developments are likely to extend beyond the health sector and become established over the long term, for example, by accentuating the scope of existing systems or those being tested (Ulbricht and Yeung 2021), facial recognition and real-time surveillance systems in mobility zones (e.g., train stations, airports), and even more large-scale projects, such as China's social credit system.

From algorithmic surveillance to citizen vigilance, does the COVID-19 pandemic reflect a change in the degree or nature of control and relations between the rulers and the ruled? This remains an open question.

Conclusion

Whether we are talking about digital platforms' proliferation into our daily lives, an infodemic, surveillance, or the control of health-related informants, through technological developments or whistleblowing, current dynamics are shedding new light on issues that lie at the very heart of our democratic societies. On the one hand, tracking applications more broadly raise the question of the secondary uses of sensitive—even anonymized—data collected and processed in the name of an emergency from forms of public–private partnerships and digital platforms. Thus, over and above the necessary oversight mechanisms, it is quite simply the destruction of data—in this case relating to health, interactions, and individual movements—collected in such a context that must take precedence to avoid any misuse for commercial or political purposes. On the other hand, the renewed forms of whistleblowing that have been witnessed, whether in response to official appeals from government representatives or not, call into question our civic-minded relationship and what it should encompass.

Notes

1.   As of July 2023, Twitter became X.
2.   See *Canada's Communications Future: Time to Act*, a report by the Broadcasting and Telecommunications Legislative Review Panel, which makes concrete

proposals for subjecting platforms to legal obligations to better control their operations, and for renewing the role of oversight bodies such as the Canadian Radio-television and Telecommunications Commission. Government of Canada, *Canada's Communications Future: Time to Act*, January 2020, https://ised-isde. canada.ca/site/broadcasting-telecommunications-legislative-review/en/canadas-communications-future-time-act.

3.   R *v.* Zundel, [1992] 2 S.C.R. 731. See https://scc-csc.lexum.com/scc-csc/scc-csc/en/item/904/index.do.

4.   *FranceTV*, "Covid-19 : plus de six Français sur dix favorables au pass sanitaire et à la vaccination obligatoire des soignants, selon notre sondage," July 16, 2021. https://www.francetvinfo.fr/sante/maladie/coronavirus/pass-sanitaire/covid-19-plus-de-six-francais-sur-dix-favorables-au-pass-sanitaire-et-a-la-vaccination-obligatoire-des-soignants-selon-notre-sondage_4705089.html. *Journal de Montréal*, "Passeport vaccinal : 'il y a une acceptation parmi la population québécoise,'" August 10, 2021. https://www.journaldemontreal.com/2021/08/10/passeport-vaccinal-il-y-a-une-acceptation-parmi-la-population-quebecoise-1.

5.   Tremblay, Julie, 9 avril 2020, COVID-19 : Les appels des citoyens engorgent les lignes d'urgence, *Ici Radio-Canada*, https://ici.radio-canada.ca/nouvelle/1692387/coronavirus-appels-911-police-rassemblements-distanciation-regles.

References

Beaud, Olivier, and Cécile Guérin-Bargues. 2020. "L'état d'urgence sanitaire : était-il judicieux de créer un nouveau régime d'exception?" *Recueil Dalloz* 16: 891.

Bigo, Didier. 2020. "Covid-19 Tracking Apps, Or: How to Deal with a Pandemic Most Unsuccessfully." *About: Intel. European Voices on Surveillance*, June 3, 2020. https://aboutintel.eu/covid-digital-tracking/.

Brodeur, Jean-Paul, and Fabien Jobard. 2005. *Citoyens et délateurs : la délation peut-elle être civique?* Paris: Éditions Autrement.

Champeil-Desplats, Véronique. 2017. "Histoire de lumières françaises : l'état d'urgence ou comment l'exception se fond dans le droit commun sans révision constitutionnelle." *Revue interdisciplinaire d'études juridiques* 79, no. 2: 205–227. https://doi.org/10.3917/riej.079.0205.

Charon, Paul, and Vilmer, Jean Baptiste Jeangène. 2021. "Les opérations d'influence chinoises : un moment machiavélien." *Institut de Recherche Stratégique de l'École Militaire (IRSEM)*. https://www.irsem.fr/institut/actualites/rapport.html.

Crichton, Cécile. 2021a. "Le Digital Service Act, un cadre européen pour la fourniture de services en ligne." *Dalloz*, January 8, 2021. https://www.dalloz-actualite.fr/flash/digital-service-act-un-cadre-europeen-pour-fourniture-de-services-en-ligne.

——. 2021b. "Le Digital Market Act, un cadre européen pour la concurrence en ligne." *Dalloz*, January 8, 2021. https://www.dalloz-actualite.fr/flash/digital-market-act-un-cadre-europeen-pour-concurrence-en-ligne.

De Comarmond, Leïla. 2021. "Covid : feu vert du Conseil constitutionnel au pass sanitaire." *Les Echos*, August 5, 2021 https://www.lesechos.fr/economie-france/social/covid-feu-vert-du-conseil-constitutionnel-au-pass-sanitaire-1337162.

Deloire, Christophe. 2020. *Working Group on Infodemics: Policy Framework, November 2020*. Forum on Information and Democracy. https://informationdemocracy.org/wp-content/uploads/2020/11/ForumID_Report-on-infodemics_101120.pdf.

Delouche-Bertolasi, Charles. 2020. "Confinement : le préfet de Seine-et-Marne réquisitionne les gardes-chasses puis recule." *Libération*, April 9, 2020. https://www.liberation.fr/france/2020/04/09/confinement-le-prefet-de-seine-et-marne-requisitionne-les-gardes-chasses-puis-recule_1784739/.

DiResta, Renée. 2018. "Computational Propaganda: If You Make It Trend, You Make It True." *The Yale Review* 106, no. 4 (October): 12–29. https://yalereview.yale.edu/computational-propaganda.

Henrotin, Joseph. 2018. "Le concept de guerre hybride." *Revue Stratégique* 3 (120): 207–211.

Kauffmann, Alexandre. 2020. "Avec le coronavirus, le retour des 'corbeaux.'" *Le Monde*, April 10, 2020. https://www.lemonde.fr/societe/article/2020/04/10/avec-le-coronavirus-le-retour-des-corbeaux_6036165_3224.html.

McIntyre, Lee. 2018. *Post-Truth*. Cambridge: The MIT Press.

Merton, Robert K. 2016. "The Self-Fulfilling Prophecy." *The Antioch Review* 74, no. 3 (Summer): 504–521.

Morozov, Evgeny. 2014. *To Save Everything, Click Here: The Folly of Technological Solutionism*. New York: Public Affairs.

Noble, Safiya Umoja. 2018. *Algorithms of Oppression. How Search Engines Reinforce Racism*. New York: New York University Press.

Rémy, Jean-Philippe. 2020. "Coronavirus : à Johannesburg, en temps de confinement, vive la délation!" *Le Monde*, April 9, 2020. https://www.lemonde.fr/afrique/article/2020/04/09/coronavirus-a-johannesburg-en-temps-de-confinement-vive-la-delation_6036048_3212.html.

Sheptycki, James. 2020. "The Politics of Policing a Pandemic Panic." *Australian & New Zealand Journal of Criminology* 53, no. 2: 157–173. https://doi.org/10.1177/0004865820925861.

Tobelem, Boran. 2021, "Covid-19 : dans quels pays d'Europe un pass sanitaire est-il en vigueur ?" *Touteleurope.eu*, September 2, 2021. https://www.touteleurope.eu/societe/covid-19-dans-quels-pays-d-europe-un-pass-sanitaire-national-est-il-en-vigueur/.

Tréguer, Félix. 2020. "Gestion techno-policière d'une crise sanitaire." *Sciences Po Centre de recherches internationales*, May 6, 2020. https://www.sciencespo.fr/ceri/fr/content/gestion-techno-policiere-d-une-crise-sanitaire.

Ulbricht, Lena and Karen Yeung. 2021. "Algorithmic Regulation: A Maturing Concept for Investigating Regulation *of* and *through* Algorithms", *Regulation and Governance*, 16, no. 1: 3–22.

Van Dijck, Jose. 2013. *The Culture of Connectivity: A Critical History of Social Media*. Oxford: Oxford University Press.

Zuboff, Shoshana. 2019. *The Age of Surveillance Capitalism. The Fight for a Human Future at the New Frontier of Power*. London: Profile Books.

CHAPTER 5

Environment and Climate Change

Pierre-Olivier Pineau, Maya Jegen, Erick Lachapelle,
Justin Leroux, and Hamish van der Ven

The pandemic is just one of the adverse effects humans have had on the planet. According to scientists, humanity's increasing proximity to the habitat of wild animals increases the likelihood of a virus, such as COVID-19, passing from an animal species to ours. In this chapter, we give an overview of environmental issues and their key features, then describe how COVID-19 could affect not only our individual actions but also the economy and governance. We conclude with a series of progressive and pragmatic ideas for how to help human societies strike an ecological balance that will ensure their sustainable development.

Pre-pandemic

Environmental problems are among the planet's greatest existential threats. Climate change is exacerbating extreme heat, drought, and forest fires, and dwindling water supplies. According to experts, we have barely a decade left to limit global warming to 1.5°C. Exceeding this threshold increases the likelihood of the above-mentioned phenomena, to which society will have to adapt as a matter of urgency. The *Global Environment Outlook*—the sixth edition of the United Nations Environment Programme's (UNEP) flagship report (Ekins et al. 2019)—shows that regularly updated evidence points to worrying trends. From air to biodiversity, oceans and coasts to land, soil, and freshwater—climate change is affecting them all.

The emission of particulate pollution is the main air-related issue. Air pollution, smog, ozone, greenhouse gases (GHGs), and persistent organic pollutants (POPs) have direct and indirect impacts on human health, food safety, ecosystems, and material goods. International treaties have effectively combatted ozone-depleting substances and certain POPs. However, new chemical threats linked to POPs are creating cause for concern. Moreover, while air quality is improving in many wealthy countries, many emerging economies, which are experiencing significant population growth, are suffering from poor air quality. The economic and social costs of pollution (e.g., public health and direct and indirect economic losses) are in the billions of dollars.

The trend in anthropogenic GHGs—primarily carbon dioxide (CO_2), methane (CH_4), and nitrous oxide (N_2O)—is also unequivocal: the growth in their emissions accelerated from 2000 to 2010 (see Figure 1). There is no sign of a reversal of this trend in the annual balances, which explains the rising concentration of these gases in the atmosphere. According to current climate projections, maintaining this trend until 2100 would result in average global warming of at least 3.5°C—far above the Paris Agreement targets of 2°C and 1.5°C

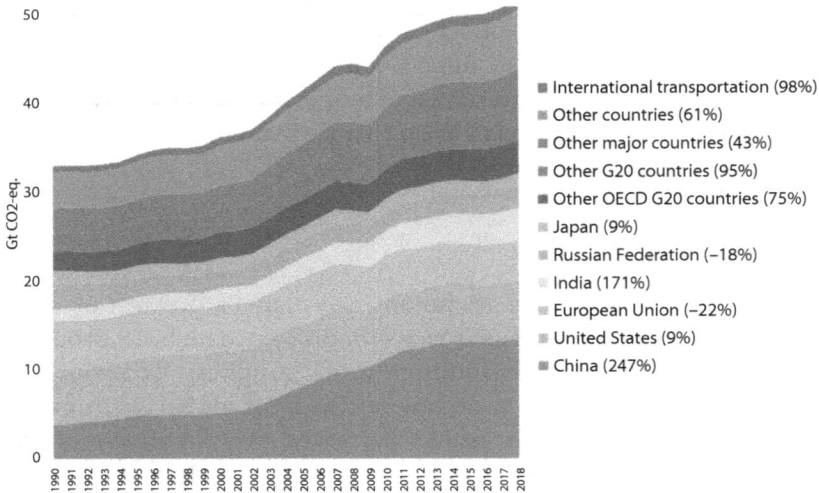

Figure 5.1. Global greenhouse gas emissions by country, 1990 to 2018, in billion tonnes of CO2 equivalent (Gt CO2-eq).

Source: Olivier and Peters, "Trends in Global CO2 and Total Greenhouse Gas Emissions", Report no. 4068. PBL Netherlands Environmental Assessment Agency, The Hague, 2019.

(UNEP 2019). Such a temperature rise would make human life impossible in many parts of the world.

According to the UNEP report, biodiversity (i.e., the degree of variability in living species) is in crisis because of the decline in the number of species observed in all natural environments. This is reflected in a decline in ecosystems' capacity to provide valuable services to all living things. These services include producing renewable natural resources, such as forests, agriculture, air and water purification, and erosion control.

In the context of COVID-19, it is important to note that the growing human population is diminishing and destroying natural habitats and biodiversity, which, in turn, brings humans closer to wild ecosystems and organisms. This proximity increases the risk of contagion (or spillover): studies indicate that zoonotic diseases (those transmitted from animals to humans) are becoming increasingly common and pose a threat to global health, the global economy, and global security.

Genetic diversity is essential for adapting to changing living conditions on Earth. As climate change alters these conditions, the loss of biodiversity has a direct impact on ecosystems' ability to adapt.

Oceans cover the majority of the Earth's surface and provide nearly half of all humans with a significant proportion of the protein they consume. They are also essential to the functioning of terrestrial ecosystems. The bleaching of coral reefs—caused primarily by ocean acidification—on which many marine ecosystems depend, overfishing, mercury accumulation, and plastic waste pollution are worrying trends that are all becoming worse. Additional problems include sandpit quarrying on marine coasts and the human noise that disturbs the marine environment. Deep-water mine development is also likely to exacerbate these phenomena.

The UNEP report stresses that agriculture and deforestation are the main land- and soil-related environmental issues, with environmental pressure keeping pace with the food needs of the planet's inhabitants. The increase in the consumption of animal proteins—the production of which requires large swaths of cereal crops—poses a challenge: as the population increases, arable land is depleted. At the same time, erosion, salinization, compaction, contamination, declining organic matter, forest fires, and overgrazing are all contributing to a deterioration in soil quality and—consequently—yield. In some regions, desertification and melting permafrost exacerbate these problems. The quantity and quality of freshwater are also declining sharply on a global scale, despite the fact that it is essential to both various ecosystems and human health. Environmental pressure is increasing as a result of agriculture, industry and energy production, and population growth.

The global nature of the COVID-19 pandemic means that it has had a significant environmental impact. While the radical reduction in the movement of people in 2020 considerably improved our carbon footprint and air quality—at least temporarily—the use of personal protective equipment (including single-use gloves and surgical masks) has led to a considerable increase in plastic waste. The use of digital services (or streaming) for entertainment and remote work also increases energy demand and, therefore, leads to increased pollution.

Why Is It So Difficult to Solve Environmental Problems?

The environmental situation is well documented and, despite the few uncertainties that remain, the trends are indisputable. It is not a lack of scientific knowledge that prevents us from tackling environmental problems, especially as several solutions for reducing or eliminating certain types of pollution are already being considered. These require technological developments and behavioural changes, and their implementation is hampered as much by the nature of the environmental problems as by psychological, institutional, and political factors.

The Double Tragedy

The so-called "super wicked" character of many environmental problems is one barrier to implementing an effective strategy. Super wicked problems have four traits: time pressure, the fact that the issue is caused by the same people who need to solve it, the need for a central authority—which is weak or non-existent—to solve the problem, and the irrational tendency to focus on the present instead of the future (Levin et al. 2012). These super wicked problems are so-called because they have no obvious solution, making them doubly devastating. First, our democratic institutions tend to devise policies that meet short-term expectations and fail to consider the urgency of the problems. Second, individual rationality comes up against the need for decisive collective action—in the so-called "tragedy of the commons," individual incentives are far too diffuse to convince people to act in favour of the common good. These two tragedies, which are tied to the very nature of environmental problems, can give rise to a sort of fatalism.

Psychological Distance

Psychological distance is the second barrier limiting the implementation of potential solutions. This term—which refers to an individual's cognitive distance from future objects or events—has four dimensions: social, temporal, spatial, and experiential (Liberman and Trope 2008). This psychological distance can be significant in the context of increasing urbanization and economic dematerialization, and it can hinder individual commitment and collective mobilization to combat climate change.

The concept's social dimension relates to how difficult it is to make a link between environmental problems, the polluters who cause them, and the people affected by them. Often, the people who create the problems are also those who are least susceptible to their impacts, so environmental problems affect only "others." If an individual is not worried, then there is less urgency to act. The temporal dimension relates to the gap between the present and the future. Problems like climate change usually have long-term impacts. Therefore, immediate action seems disconnected from its ultimate purpose, which will only materialize in the distant future. With temporal distance, immediate action and its associated costs seem irrational, as the benefits can only be reaped in the long term. Furthermore, people's (urban) homes may be a long way from the places most hard hit by environmental problems—oceans, tropical forests, and the countries of the Global South. The spatial dimension of psychological distance also leads people to feel detached from the urgency of the situation. Lastly, the experiential dimension refers to individuals' real-life experience of the problem. In a world of growing dematerialization and virtual reality, humanity is increasingly removed from the natural environment. Similarly, uncertainty over the future impacts of extreme weather conditions and about the extent to which human activity is responsible creates another type of distance between environmental problems and potential solutions.

These different dimensions of psychological distance foster a disengaged attitude to environmental problems. Because these challenges require people to make lifestyle changes—and to avoid cognitive dissonance—the general population prefers to ignore the problems and carry on with their regular behaviours and habits. In a way, psychological distance justifies this avoidance.

Imperfect Governance

Despite environmental issues having been on the political radar for over half a century, in the face of scientific evidence of the urgent need for action, the results have been disappointing. The very nature of the super wicked problems involved, as well as the notion of psychological distance, explain why governments find it difficult to develop policies that meet long-term objectives. The in-depth reforms the complexity of environmental problems require are not compatible with the election cycle. Psychological distance is a problem not only for citizens, but also for politicians, which only exacerbates the tragedy of the commons.

Over the past fifty years, several environmental institutions have been created at the international, national, and subnational levels. For example, UNEP is great at documenting problems, but it has a very limited scope for action. The United Nations Framework Convention on Climate Change began a process that incorporates the Kyoto Protocol and the Paris Agreement. Both help keep the climate issue on the global political agenda but do little to bring us closer to CO_2 reduction targets (e.g., those advocated by the scientific community).

There are still many obstacles to the efforts required to achieve a more ambitious international climate regime. According to the countries of the Global South, industrialized countries should bear the costs of decarbonization and climate change adaptation because of their historical responsibility for the current problems. In addition, the Global South faces the challenge of reducing energy poverty within their borders while struggling with limited financial and other resources. Industrialized countries believe that all nation-states must make firm commitments, respecting the principle of sovereign equality of states, as GHG emissions are expected to be very high in the Global South. Furthermore, the growing economic rivalry between China and the United States—which, between them, account for over 40 percent of global emissions—undermines the goal of preventing global temperatures from rising to the 2°C limit. As it stands, climate policy risks becoming a bargaining chip in the balance of power between the two hegemonic countries.

Without a central authority at the global level, it is difficult to align different interests or sanction harmful behaviour. International environmental institutions are fragmented. Moreover, while non-state actors are partially filling the void left by states and market forces are increasingly used to counter environmental problems, this type of governance has yet to prove effective.

Coordination and cooperation problems arise nationally both vertically and horizontally. The first relates to federalism, since environmental objectives and how to achieve them must be negotiated by the various levels of government. Municipal governments are also involved, even if they lack the resources to act. Horizontally—and in a distributional policy logic—coordination can pose challenges, as government departments and agencies have differing priorities, reflecting their mandate to promote the interests of those who contribute to climate change.

The Pandemic's Environmental Impact

Against the backdrop of this multidimensional environmental crisis, the COVID-19 pandemic has had a variety of impacts. While many have called for a green economic recovery and an acceleration of the energy transition to combat climate change, environmental regulations are also being relaxed to facilitate investment projects. In this section, we look at how the pandemic could affect—positively or negatively—individual, economic, and institutional environmental trajectories.

Individual Priorities

Lockdowns and social distancing could lead to individuals adopting new attitudes, changing people's psychological distance from certain issues. The pandemic has highlighted many social inequalities and the poor quality of services certain social groups are offered (e.g., older adults in long-term care facilities or private seniors' residences). This will hopefully lead to greater solidarity, enabling the necessary investments in social and environmental policy. By highlighting societal shortcomings, the pandemic could help our societies become more proactive, less vulnerable, and more resilient.

From another perspective, the inward-looking nature of lockdowns could provoke a diametrically opposed reaction. Individuals could choose to prioritize their immediate safety and comfort, thus spending more, for example on larger homes, ideally with swimming pools (to compensate for a lack of access to municipal facilities), and on larger vehicles to avoid public transport and feel safe. Despite the economic uncertainties the pandemic caused, these trends are already being observed on the market, where consumers are turning to the purchase of single-family homes and additional personal vehicles. Continuing with this scenario would compound the tragedy of the commons by increasing GHG emissions through our individual behaviours.

Economic Pressures

Because of the economic slowdown and restrictions on the movement of people at the start of the pandemic, pollution fell. However, this was short-lived and, as the economy recovered, pollution once again increased. Nevertheless, could the pandemic prove to be a turning point in terms of pollution?

On the one hand, new pandemic-related practices that would reduce the environmental footprint of human activities could be extended. For example, a telework-induced reduction in the need to travel would significantly decrease GHG emissions. In addition, local production would help reduce transport-related pollution and strengthen solidarity with local workers, thereby reducing the psychological distance—especially its spatial aspect—between producer and consumer. Improving self-sufficiency through local production would strengthen our societal resilience. Furthermore, economic recovery could be accompanied by "green" investments (e.g., in infrastructure) that take into account the limits of ecosystems. In the medium term, fluctuations in oil prices could accelerate the decline of the fossil fuel industry and guide investors toward more promising sectors, such as renewable energy or more energy-efficient equipment.

On the other hand, the end of the pandemic could lead to a sustained increase in pollution, as was the case after the 2007–2008 economic crisis. The desire for rapid recovery could lead to reliance on the familiar formulas that contributed to the above-described environmental damage. These are well-established economic players—often seen as structural to national economies—that drive investment in traditional sectors, such as oil and gas or road construction. Relying on road infrastructure, cash injections to boost consumption, and other economic growth plans based on past practices could further reinforce negative environmental trends. For example, in the wake of the 2007–2008 financial crisis, the U.S. government bailed out the auto industry, which took advantage of the situation to increase its production of gas-guzzling models. Government action thus indirectly supported the growth of GHG emissions in the transportation sector. As we emerge from the pandemic, there is a fear that economic pressures will take precedence over environmental considerations.

Governance Overhaul

COVID-19 showed that governments are capable of acting swiftly, declaring a state of emergency that often centralizes power and restricts economic and individual freedoms. Will crisis governance have lasting impacts?

It is true that the pandemic could inspire reforms and serve as justification for much-needed investments, particularly in the field of public health, which includes environmental parameters. These reforms and investments would make societies more resilient in the face of health or environmental crises that scientists believe will occur in the future. These reforms should address the coordination issues mentioned above, between different departments (e.g., transportation, energy, and the environment), but also between different levels of government.

However, it is feared that the concentration of power that we experienced during the pandemic will become a permanent fixture, to the detriment of democratic processes. As governments unblock unprecedented financial resources to revive the economy post-lockdown while relaxing certain measures (e.g., consultation or environmental assessment requirements), environmental assessment and citizen consultation procedures risk being undermined.

Internationally, the pandemic has overshadowed and slowed global climate governance progress while offering glimmers of hope. COP26 in Glasgow was postponed, delaying an important international climate summit at a critical point in history. The pandemic also interrupted the momentum of the global Fridays For Future movement, which had mobilized a generation of young activists. Yet, it has had an interesting effect on the private sector, leading to renewed interest in global supply chains. Many companies are looking to relocate their production and to better understand their supply chain and associated partners. It is perhaps this improved communication across global supply chains that has prompted companies such as Unilever and Logitech to better understand the carbon footprint of their products and to assess each one, throughout its life cycle.

Avoiding a Sad Return to Reality

To protect the environment and counter climate change, we need to take measures that are both cross-cutting—to change practices structurally in all sectors—and specific to the major impact sectors. Here, we look at specific measures in land-use planning, industry, transportation, and construction; due to a lack of space, we have omitted agriculture from our discussion.

While some of the proposed measures are a direct result of lockdowns (large-scale telework is possible!), most are designed to avoid a sad return to reality while taking advantage of the crisis to make a change. The pandemic is a concrete reminder of the importance of preparing for crises and mitigating their risks. Epidemiologists have long alerted governments to the risk of a pandemic, as have environmental and pandemic scientists. If there is one lesson to be learned, it is to not give in to the temptation of short-termism (Ness 2020).

Cross-Cutting Measures

Scrapping Pollution Subsidies and Implementing Ecotaxation

As costly stimulus and aid packages are being deployed to counter the economic crisis, governments must put an end to their practice of systematically subsidizing polluters—which is still commonplace—particularly in the oil and gas sector (direct and indirect subsidies). Scrapping the various forms of tax relief for polluters must go hand in hand with progressive and widespread ecotaxation: in a context of unprecedented public indebtedness, taxing polluting activities will generate financial resources that will improve natural environments and reduce the tax burden.[1] On an international scale, this could be part of a debate on government assistance, some of which is already prohibited by international standards, and on tax competition.

Providing Continuing Education to Support the Global Energy Transition

The COVID-19 pandemic highlighted how vulnerable many national economies are, particularly in terms of employment. Similarly, climate change and the transition to a low-carbon society require investing in a more agile workforce. To ensure that all those affected by the economic impacts of the COVID-19 pandemic and the economic transition to a low-carbon society can return to work, as well as to ensure universal access to the acquisition of new skills, major efforts must be made in the continuing education sector.

As education becomes more globalized, educational institutions must improve their offerings and facilitate the renewal of individual expertise to simplify work-related changes and mitigate the insecurity people feel about the economic transition. Practically speaking, governments should invest more in institutions that offer vocational training and offer tax incentives for continuing education and going back to school, particularly in fields related to the energy transition. In this respect, the solution involves — in part — international cooperation in the fields of education and vocational training.

Sector-Specific Measures

Land-Use Planning: Protecting Ecosystems

The cohabitation of human societies and other living species is all too often to the detriment of the latter. Humans' imperialism over the environment must be contained to rebalance ecosystems, which are essential to human survival. As the short-term pressure to individualize homes and transportation grows, resisting urban sprawl and further protecting agricultural and natural areas — both in developed countries and elsewhere in the world — will be critical. As recognized by the Convention on Biological Diversity, forms of urbanization and biodiversity are intimately linked.

Developing Stimulus Plans in Line with International Environmental Commitments

The scale of the economic stimulus plans was an opportunity worth seizing, and hopefully it is not squandered. In Canada — as elsewhere—government assistance to industry should be conditional on establishing a decarbonization plan and achieving ambitious GHG reduction targets. Such a plan would provide a roadmap of actions to take to decarbonize corporate operations. Some countries seem to be choosing this option as a way out of the health crisis. For example, the Austrian government decided to make any bailout of Austrian Airlines conditional on it achieving climate targets; the plan is to reduce short-haul flights and increase cooperation with rail companies. Similarly, Sweden tied its public funding of Scandinavian Airlines to quantitative targets in line with the Paris Agreement's 1.5°C objective. Such eco-conditionality would also be desirable for loans and grants from major international institutions, such as the World Bank and the International Monetary Fund.

However, not every industry should qualify for government assistance. Just as companies that place funds in tax havens are no longer eligible for government bailouts in France, Belgium, and Denmark, industries that actively undermine a country's Paris Climate Accord commitments should also be prevented from receiving COVID-19 bailouts. For example, the coal industry is in structural decline and should not be kept alive with public funds. In return for public support for high-carbon companies, governments should be offered shares in them. They should also have the authority to define and implement aggressive carbon mitigation policies. Such plans would avoid saving large industries without structural transformation and repeating the mistakes made after the 2007–2008 financial crisis.

Nevertheless, there is a key lesson to be learned from the financial- and banking-sector reforms made in the wake of that crisis. At the time, governments had imposed guidelines on the financial sector to prevent the recurrence of excesses such as the subprime crisis, which occurred when the market for non-bank asset-backed commercial paper collapsed. Similarly, environmental conditions should be imposed on COVID-related stimulus investments.

Transportation: Rethinking Local and International Travel

One major outcome of the 2020 lockdown is that, for a significant number of jobs, telework became possible on a large scale. The "return to normal" must consider these changes and standardize virtual international meetings. This will reduce transportation-related GHG emissions, and the travel time saved will boost productivity.

A rise in related electricity demand—somewhat less problematic in areas which can source clean electricity—is to be expected.

Rethinking travel also means developing active transportation methods, such as walking, cycling, and public transit. Internationally, rail transportation infrastructure—particularly electric—for both people and goods should be prioritized. Rail transportation not only has a smaller footprint and is much more energy efficient than road transportation, but it is also a structuring factor, as it encourages the densification of inhabited areas, protecting land and connecting areas. The imposition of kilometre-based taxes proportional to vehicle power and weight, as well as parking taxes, would be a strong behaviour-changing incentive and would generate revenue to fund alternative solutions.

The pandemic led to a radical decline in air transportation—a sector that had been growing strongly previously and that already contributes around 2 percent of human activity-related CO_2 emissions and 3 percent of fossil fuel-related emissions. In the space of a few months, the cancellation of conventions and the reduction in international tourism and business travel positively—but extremely modestly—impacted climate change. Rather than subsidizing aircraft manufacturers' comeback, the growth of this type of transportation must be curbed. To this end, a highly structured approach would involve developing rail transportation between cities, making it more attractive than air travel by offering a superior time-comfort-cost combination.

Construction: Sharing Best Practices

One cross-cutting measure for protecting the environment and combatting climate change is workforce agility and continuing education. The construction industry stands to benefit from this, as building greener housing requires a skilled workforce of tradespeople and architects trained in energy-efficient housing standards, such as low-energy and passive houses, and zero-energy and positive-energy buildings.

Socially speaking, housing inequalities have dramatic impacts on people's quality of life and health. As the COVID-19 pandemic clearly demonstrated, infection and death rates were much higher in low-income neighbourhoods with high population density and poor-quality apartments. A progressive housing policy could foster social inclusion and equity while reducing the ecological and energy foot-print. For example, passive buildings—designed to avoid an active heating system—can reduce energy consumption by over 80 percent. These techniques are well known and widespread in several countries, notably in Germany and in the Scandinavian countries. The pandemic did not curb the global spread of ideas, through which building codes and energy-efficient standards and practices could be updated in line with global best practices. At the very least, measuring and disclosing the energy performance of buildings should become mandatory, to raise awareness of the potential for improvements in this sector.

Conclusion

Not only are the number and scale of environmental problems—driven by climate change—challenging, but their very "super wicked" nature and the psychological distance that blinds us have made solving them impossible until now. COVID-19 can accelerate environmental damage or—on the contrary—create an opportunity to trigger the societal transformation required to improve the situation. The risk of the former is significant. However, the pandemic has upended our lives and shown that scientists' warnings about the threat of a pandemic was not a false alarm.

Time is running out to take the warnings on environmental and climate change seriously. The measures put forth in this chapter aim to steer our society towards a more balanced relationship with the natural environment. This requires individual, economic, and institutional changes to make our lifestyles compatible with the limits of our ecosystems. In practical terms, this means considering the life cycle of products and services; reducing, reusing, and recycling (3Rs) resources in a circular economy; and adding the fourth "R"—refuse! A more sustainable and just world would be more resilient in the next crisis.

Notes

1. Ecotaxation measures involve charging economic players (businesses and indi-viduals, in particular) for certain activities to modify their behaviour. These measures have proved effective in a number of areas, including waste manage-ment and the reduction of vehicle traffic and GHG emissions.

References

Ekins, Paul, Joyeeta Gupta, and Pierre Boileau, eds. 2019. *Global Environment Outlook: Healthy Planet, Healthy People*. Cambridge: Cambridge University Press. https://doi.org/10.1017/9781108627146.

Levin, Kelly, Benjamin Cashore, Steven Bernstein, and Graeme Auld. 2012. "Overcoming the Tragedy of Super Wicked Problems: Constraining Our Future Selves to Ameliorate Global Climate Change." *Policy Sciences* 45, no. 2 (June): 123–152. https://doi.org/10.1007/s11077-012-9151-0.

Liberman, Nira, and Yaacov Trope. 2008. "The Psychology of Transcending the Here and Now." *Science* 322, no. 5905 (November): 1201–1205. https://www.science.org/doi/10.1126/science.1161958.

Ness, Ryan. 2020. "Prior Preparation Pays Off." Canadian Climate Institute, June 23, 2020. https://climatechoices.ca/prior-preparation-pays-off/.

Olivier, Jos, and Jeroen Peters. 2020. *Trends in Global CO2 and Total Greenhouse Gas Emissions. 2019 Report*. The Hague: PBL Netherlands Environmental Assessment Agency.

UNEP (United Nations Environment Programme). 2019. *Emissions Gap Report 2019*. Nairobi: UNEP. https://wedocs.unep.org/bitstream/handle/20.500.11822/30797/EGR2019.pdf.

CHAPTER 6

Peace and Security

Theodore McLauchlin, Sarah-Myriam Martin-Brûlé,
María Martín de Almagro Iniesta,
Lee Seymour, and Marie-Joëlle Zahar

On 23 March 2020, United Nations (UN) Secretary-General António Guterres issued a plea for a global ceasefire in the face of the pandemic. His statement included a reminder that even warring factions had in COVID-19 a common enemy. It then took over three months—until 1 July—for the UN Security Council's 15 Member States to take the next step and agree to a resolution calling for a 90-day global humanitarian ceasefire.

The delay illustrates a central paradox in the relationship between the pandemic and war. As Guterres argued, COVID-19 gave everyone, even bitter adversaries, reasons to cooperate. But the necessary cooperation has seemed very often to be a long way off. The pandemic strengthened the imperative to act on armed conflict. Displaced populations can be especially vulnerable to infectious diseases, and wars make it harder to secure medical care. In some places, such as Libya and Yemen, wars initially intensified during the pandemic; in others, such as in India and the United States, social conflicts have deepened and may tip toward organized violence.

However, despite the urgency, these events occurred against the backdrop of missing diplomatic leadership, strained international cooperation, and rising tensions among the world's most powerful states. By the time a bickering United States and China agreed to the precise language of the Security Council resolution, parties to the conflicts in Yemen and Colombia who had initially signed on to the proposal had already resumed fighting (International Crisis Group 2020a).

COVID-19 has evolved rapidly, and its many unknowns make prediction difficult. Our effort in this chapter is to draw out general trends in the emergence and management of armed conflicts, both within countries and between them. We first discuss the key trends in conflict before the pandemic. We then move on to the impact of COVID-19 on the emergence and severity of armed conflicts and on conflict management by the international community. Next, we discuss how pandemic response can make conflict impacts worse. Throughout, we illustrate how the pandemic affects peace and security through its economic shocks, its restrictions on face-to-face contact and travel, and how it seems to push aside so many other priorities. Through these effects, paradoxically, COVID-19 brings both more reasons to cooperate but also, very often, more sources of mistrust.

It is also important not to overestimate the impact of COVID-19 on international peace and security. The war in Ukraine, instead, has dominated the global attention since February 2022, and the consequences of this war have been and will continue to be profound across multiple domains: food insecurity, arms control, defense policy, NATO cohesion, UN diplomacy, and the risk of conflict over Taiwan, to name a few. However, the pandemic *has* played a role in exacerbating existing mistrust internationally, suggesting that its effects will be manifest in multiple security fronts.

War in the Before Time

The level of armed conflict looked increasingly discouraging before 2020. Until a few years prior, the global count of armed conflicts from projects like the Uppsala Conflict Data Program (UCDP) had suggested that the world was rising to the challenge of war (e.g., Goldstein 2011). Though the disintegration of Yugoslavia and the Soviet Union combined with state collapse to produce wars in places such as Bosnia, Chechnya, Somalia, and Rwanda, a combination of military victories, peace agreements, robust peacekeeping, and international cooperation sharply curtailed these wars thereafter. In the post-Cold War world, with a few notable exceptions such as Ethiopia-Eritrea, India-Pakistan, or the invasions of Iraq (and now the invasion of Ukraine), interstate war has been a remarkably rare event. Though less dramatically, war within countries (intrastate conflict) also declined after hitting a peak in 1991, dropping from 51 to roughly 35 active intrastate wars through much of the 2000s (Petterson, Högbladh, and Öberg 2019).

These promising downward trends reversed sharply from 2012, however, with 2017 surpassing the previous record with 53 armed conflicts. Much of this increase was driven by the Islamic State (ISIS) and its affiliates. The risk of interstate war also returned to the forefront of the international agenda with Russia's 2014 incursions in Ukraine, the 2017-2018 nuclear crisis in the Korean Peninsula, rising tensions over territorial disputes between China and its neighbours, and new developments in strategic technology such as hypersonic missiles. The number of fatalities in armed conflicts hit a bloody summit in 2014, driven by the Syrian civil war, though it has declined since (Petterson, Högbladh, and Öberg 2019). The average annual number of deaths from conflict thus increased from 55,000 in 2004–2009 to 70,000 for 2007–2012, worldwide, according to the most recent *Global Burden of Armed Violence* report. At the same time, however, this represented only about 13.8 percent of the world's total of violent deaths, some 508,000 per year in the latter period (Geneva Declaration Secretariat 2015). They are far from the seven to fifteen million deaths attributable to COVID-19.

Violence of all kinds has pushed millions to flee. During the 1990s and 2000s, roughly 40 million people were forcibly displaced. With a sharp increase from 2013 onward, that figure doubled to 79.5 million in 2019 according to the United Nations High Commissioner for Refugees (UNHCR), with conflict zones like Syria, Afghanistan, South Sudan, and Myanmar as four of the five leading countries of origin (Venezuela is in second place), though many flee violence outside of war. The vast majority of those forcibly displaced end up in neighbouring countries, with 85 percent of them hosted in developing countries such as Turkey, Pakistan, and Uganda (UNHCR 2020). The war in Ukraine has displaced some 6.3 million refugees, about 15 percent of the prewar population.

Contemporary armed conflicts often have features that make them difficult to resolve. To begin, today's civil wars are highly internationalized, with UCDP data suggesting that outside players have deployed troops to as many as 30 percent of conflicts in recent years. Wars in Syria, Yemen, and Libya, which are overlaid with competition among regional powers like Iran, Saudi Arabia, Turkey, and Egypt, and a growing rift between Russia and the West, are emblematic. But by no means is this a solely Middle Eastern phenomenon as illustrated by Russia's involvement in Ukraine between 2014 and its full-scale invasion in February 2022, or the long-standing involvement of Sudan and Chad in the Central African Republic. A second and related feature is the fragmentation and multiplication of actors in today's wars. The fractured Syrian opposition and its hundreds of armed actors is the most extreme example. A third feature of these wars is that they often have a religious dimension, most prominently the involvement of transnational jihadist groups such as ISIS or al-Qaeda with links to locally rooted groups such as Boko Haram, the Taliban, or al-Shabab (Walter 2017). In short, contemporary civil conflicts have a large number of players with many agendas, many of which admit little compromise. Arriving at negotiated settlements and maintaining ceasefires in these circumstances is challenging at best.

Also prior to 2020, several worrying geopolitical changes were emerging. A truculent, isolationist United States under President Trump was hamstrung by domestic political polarization. Washington thus abdicated the leadership role it has occupied since 1945. Europe has been likewise focused inward, struggling to manage violence on its periphery in Ukraine, Libya, and Syria while it concentrates on hardening borders and negotiating the future of the European project. If the war in Ukraine led to a course correction and a revitalization of allied cooperation on both sides of the Atlantic, it is not clear how long it will last.

Russia's invasion was also the culmination of a long increase in tension among great powers. Russia had attempted to reassert power by developing new missile systems, carrying out bold and brutal interventions in Syria, and expanding its presence in the Middle East and Sub-Saharan Africa, exploiting the vacuum left by Western powers. China, meanwhile, has concentrated on its increasingly aggressive posture toward Taiwan, its regional territorial disputes in the South China Sea and with India, consolidating its grasp on restive Hong Kong, implementing draconian measures on the Uighur population in Xinjiang, and cementing economic relations through its Belt and Road Initiative. Competition between the United States and China had been increasing before the pandemic, with damaging trade disputes and bitter conflicts about cybersecurity and espionage. Regional powers have had new opportunities to flex muscles, fulfill geopolitical ambitions, and distract from domestic political problems, driving violence in places like Libya, Yemen, and Syria.

These trends appear to herald a greater likelihood of international conflict and make it harder to manage wars around the world. The United States and Russia have dismantled key arms control agreements like the Intermediate-Range Nuclear Forces Treaty, and the United States unilaterally withdrew from the nuclear weapons accord with Iran. Disagreements between Russia and the West even before 2022 prevented the UN Security Council from taking meaningful action on Syria. Efforts at preventing conflicts before they begin have had some significant under-the-radar successes in recent years, often with regional organizations like the Economic Community of West African States (ECOWAS) and the UN working in concert (Brubaker and Druet 2020). But because the United States cut its contribution, the UN peacekeeping budget was already in decline in 2019–2020, before the pandemic. Diplomatic resources around the world have been increasingly stretched thin between multiple, ongoing crises.

On the (Socially Distanced) March: COVID-19 and Armed Conflict

Then COVID-19 arrived. How has it affected armed conflict around the world, and what are its likely short-run and long-run consequences for these armed conflicts?

Start with international conflicts. On the one hand, the influential scholar Barry Posen (2020) argued compellingly that COVID-19 makes aggression by one state against another even less attractive than it was before. Economic hardship leaves states without the money to spend on aggression. It is also hard to run an active army or navy on a battle footing under social distancing. To Posen, rational states should be more inclined, not less, to avoid conflict in the world after: the common interest in maintaining peace is strong. While the Russian invasion of Ukraine seems to belie this hypothesis, it is noteworthy that the pandemic may have undermined the Russian war effort through: disruptions in training, military resources committed to public health, reduced operations at logistics hubs and depots, and economic problems affecting defense industries (Mittal 2022). COVID-19 should have induced more caution in Moscow than it did.

In line with the thesis that the pandemic can drive peace, we have indeed seen cooperative international gestures between rivals. Some Gulf states, for example, have extended humanitarian assistance to Iran, one of the early COVID-19 hotspots (Rozen 2020). More generally, states have seen that there are opportunities to advance their international influence not by military deployments or interventions, but by providing medical equipment and coordinating global vaccine research.

One might therefore expect cooperation to continue. However, the pandemic has also generated risks of worsened international tensions. It has played into and exacerbated existing mistrust and led to opportunities for states to take advantage of each other. Though Russian-Western tension has been especially dramatic, the clearest instance of the impact of COVID is in the all-important U.S.-China relationship, which has soured even more since March 2020. Officials from each have blamed the other for the pandemic, with claims ranging from the well-founded to the preposterous. China, perhaps believing that its regional and global opponents had a lot on their minds, escalated the long-running territorial disputes over the South China Sea by changing the legal status of several disputed islands and shoals, and tightened its grip on Hong Kong with a new national security law. More recently, it has rattled the sabre with Taiwan with increasing frequency and publicity. The United States, in turn, sought to isolate China, levied sanctions on some of its leaders, launched a round of embassy closings, and withdrew from the World Health Organization (WHO) for its supposedly pro-China stance. President Biden has often publicly declared American support for Taiwan in ways that seem to break with the previous policy consensus. Each side trusts the other even less than it did before the crisis, and each side is exceedingly sensitive to perceived slights.

Armed aggression between the United States and China is still unlikely. Nuclear deterrence and mutual interdependence remain and should give leaders in Beijing and Washington pause. But the United States and China can compete in other arenas, ramping up cyberattacks and economic conflict. As during the Cold War, they could continue to hobble the functioning of the UN Security Council and engage in proxy wars. By entrenching mutual mistrust, COVID-19 may have played a part in deepening a new cold war. It has often seemed since as though the risk of an armed conflict in East Asia is on the rise.

The same twin pandemic effects—a greater need for cooperation alongside worsening mistrust and unpredictable, disruptive consequences—can be seen in civil conflicts too. Armed conflicts shatter health systems, and each side has, in principle, an incentive to lay down arms to let doctors treat the sick and to reduce the movement of combatants and civilians. In countries with severe political tensions short of war, governments, oppositions, and social groups have had many reasons to cooperate in the common battle. In some instances, like Venezuela or eastern Myanmar, regimes and their opponents heeded the call to work together to fight the illness, at least temporarily (International Crisis Group 2020b). There was, on average, a decline in the frequency of battles over the course of 2020 (Pavlik 2020).

But COVID-19 created ample opportunities for conflict as well. In places where outside actors kept a fragile peace and political order, the virus weakens their willingness to do so. Powers like the United States (in Afghanistan) and France (in Mali) tired of their long-running interventions for reasons well predating the pandemic, and COVID-19 played no obvious direct role in the withdrawal of either. But the pandemic would not have helped; in particular, it would have been difficult to imagine a COVID-afflicted America deciding to escalate in Afghanistan to the extent necessary to respond to the Taliban advances of 2020.

Additionally, the pandemic created risks of new civil conflicts (Moyer and Kaplan 2020). Much like the mutual recriminations between countries, plagues often come with fear of the Other, thought to be the vector of disease, and opportunistic politicians can exploit this fear to mobilize their supporters. For example, COVID-19 came with increased attacks on Asian-Americans and on Muslims in India, where Prime Minister Narendra Modi has revoked the autonomy of Kashmir and taken a number of anti-Muslim measures since the outbreak of the pandemic.

Public health measures to deal with the pandemic became an axis of social tension as well. This debate took a dramatic turn in several countries, notably Canada and the United States, where extremists and conspiracy theorists fed on generalized frustration to forward a radical antigovernment discourse—one associated with a higher rate of acceptance of the Russian invasion of Ukraine. Indeed, the pandemic and public health response became a focal point for far-right movements in the West, an effect that seems likely to persist.

The pandemic also wrought disruptions that imperiled countries already facing fragile economic and political situations. Probably the most dramatic effect was in Ethiopia. Here, the government's decision to delay the August 2020 elections—justified with reference to the pandemic—led the government of Tigray to organize its own regional vote and touched off a political crisis and the subsequent bloody civil war. However, regional tensions long predated the pandemic, and another spark might have led to a confrontation regardless. As Comfort Ero (2021) argues, it is important not to overstate the impact of the pandemic on conflict; indeed, this can amount to blaming a disease for political failures. The same goes for the invasion of Ukraine or the war in Israel/Palestine, neither of which seems to have much to do with the pandemic.

At the same time, the disease has dramatically uneven impacts within societies. It lays bare unequal access to treatment and unequal burdens of work and economic vulnerability. While these social conflicts can often be channelled in democratic and progressive action, such as protest movements and elections, they can also take a violent course through repression and violent uprisings. Finally, pandemic response has upended politics in many countries, as leaders who were previously in good political shape now face significant internal challenges—and crack down. The United States draws together these effects: COVID-19's wildly disproportionate impact on Black Americans lay in the background when a white police officer's killing of George Floyd spurred an enormous country-wide wave of demonstrations. In turn, President Trump placed a bet on a violent "law and order" response to shore up his electoral base. In Belarus, President Lukashenko's dismissive reaction to the crisis may have added to the public's anger and its refusal to accept the results of a rigged election, and hence to the emergence of a moment of democratic mobilization and a government crackdown in response.

If the effects of COVID-19 on armed conflict are ambiguous, there appears to be no disputing that physical and structural violence have gotten worse. Under lockdown, victims of domestic abuse had very few options; they spent more time with their abusers, had few places to flee, and fewer contacts outside the home with people who can help. In some countries, calls to helplines for victims of domestic abuse increased from two to fivefold in a matter of days in spring 2020. This violence disproportionately affects women and compounds the highly gender-unequal economic effects of the illness in many societies (Azcona et al. 2020). COVID-19—on top of drought, locusts, and hurricanes—has led to increased food insecurity, as people lose livelihoods and migrate, children lose school nutrition programs, and the virus disrupts agricultural supply chains. The World Food Programme (WFP) estimated a 50 percent increase in food assistance requirements in Southern Africa compared to pre-pandemic projections. At the same time, resources for humanitarian relief have not kept pace. WFP, for example, had to scale back food relief and cash transfers to refugees in East Africa by almost 30 percent because of a cash shortfall (World Food Programme 2020). Finally, the choices around a strategy to address COVID-19 carried a high potential for structural violence, for example forcing the economically vulnerable to choose whether to work and get sick or stay home and starve. The United States, for example, used COVID-19 to justify even more restrictive asylum policies than the draconian measures it had already enacted. Those waiting to apply for asylum in the United States have suffered in makeshift camps with few services and where they are vulnerable to criminal violence. Any policy on COVID-19 and political violence needs to address this kind of insecurity at its roots.

On Mute: COVID-19 and Conflict Management

At the same time as the pandemic increased the risk of violence in some areas, it has made it harder to manage those conflicts. Above all, efforts at peace—already stretched thin before the pandemic—are likely to suffer from limited resources. Many countries may reduce the money and personnel they commit to diplomacy and peace operations as they face health crises and lingering economic disruptions at home, and worry about maintaining public order. They may adopt greater degrees of economic nationalism and reduce their assistance abroad, worsening socioeconomic conditions around the world and risking new conflicts. International diplomacy may become even more reactive than it already was, focusing increasingly limited resources on any new immediate crises and limiting the scope of conflict prevention.

Additionally, many tactics for managing international and civil conflicts depend on moving human bodies around—those of diplomats, mediators, weapons inspectors, peacekeepers, and civil society activists. Travel restrictions had a major impact on many of these activities. International diplomacy shifted to the internet, potentially making it harder to develop the informal, face-to-face ties and personal relationships that have facilitated cooperation in the past (Liechtenstein 2020). Lack of movement and health restrictions impeded inspections by the Office for the Prohibition of Chemical Weapons and the International Atomic Energy Agency, inspections that are crucial to maintaining mutual confidence and arms control. Many of these limitations have come to an end, however, and the rise of videoconferencing has possibly led to new tools as well—take, for example, the use of the tool by Ukrainian President Volodymyr Zelensky to address parliaments and international organizations worldwide.

A particularly visible impact of COVID-19 on conflict management is in peace operations, because these missions rest on large-scale movements of personnel and extensive contact with civilians. Peacekeepers bear a great deal of risk, within often complex and hostile environments and exposure to diseases. In an epidemic outbreak, the risks are exponential. Troop contributing countries (TCCs) became reluctant to let their troops face these risks. Furthermore, peacekeepers often came under no-movement orders intended to reduce the risk that they become a disease vector. Hence, personnel already on the ground in missions like South Sudan, Mali, the Central African Republic, the Democratic Republic of Congo, and Somalia had to stay long after their rotations were supposed to end, and their normal rest-and-recuperate cycles have been disrupted. These developments erode morale and efficiency, with impacts likely to linger.

Restrictions on movement also made it much harder for mission personnel to interact with local populations. Peace operations are deployed in dynamic and volatile settings with social, political, economic, and institutional vulnerabilities. These conditions make local knowledge and strong, cooperative relationships with local populations essential to success. In places of protracted conflict, such as the Central African Republic or the Democratic Republic of Congo, peacekeepers, and notably female engagement teams, conducted routine patrols and reached out to marginalized local communities. This not only reduced localized and domestic violence as well as sexual and gender-based violence, but also facilitated the gathering of invaluable intelligence that mapped out potential threats coming from armed groups and localized guerrillas. When they lack these relationships, peace operation personnel do not know when attacks are imminent, do not know what local needs are, cannot arrange the informal dialogues that are so critical to preserving peace, and make counterproductive decisions. But COVID-related requirements to work remotely and limit in-person contacts created additional hurdles for communication among staff and between the mission's staff and the local population (de Coning 2020). Though the risk has reduced, a degree of distancing seems to have emerged in a number of peace operations, and this will take time to come to an end.

Limiting in-person contact between peacekeepers and local civilians was as much for civilians' protection as for the international personnel. Some states such as South Sudan and Mali declared that they would no longer welcome troops from TCCs perceived as being the most affected by COVID-19, notably China and South Korea—the first of which is among the largest troop contriubtors (Di Razza and Sherman 2020). The fact that host states identified TCCs suggests a willingness to control the parameters of peace operations with an eye to public health. After all, UN personnel brought a devastating cholera outbreak to Haiti in 2011. Peace operations and their local partners therefore faced and may continue to face a real dilemma for future disease outbreaks: assessing how interveners could access the population and provide the required resources and medical assistance, all the while protecting civilians and their own personnel from disease transmission. At the same time, while there is a very real risk that international humanitarian workers could spread COVID-19 or future diseases, there is also a danger of rumour and of deliberate misinformation campaigns accusing peacekeepers of being the source of the virus.

Making Matters Worse

COVID-19 thus has major ramifications for armed conflict. But responses to COVID-19 can often make matters worse. In conflict-affected countries, the measures taken to control the evolution of the pandemic may have larger impacts on peace and security than COVID-19 itself. These measures do not only have medical effects, but also transform the configuration of international actors, targeted beneficiaries, and main collaborators on the ground, with potentially significant unintended consequences.

First, health programs directed at those up until now considered the most vulnerable, and in particular those directed at maternal health and infant health, have been pushed to the side. In the ongoing war in Yemen, for example, more than 30 lifesaving UN-funded humanitarian programs were due to draw down or close in spring 2020 (OCHA 2020), and support shifted toward the COVID-19 response to the detriment of basic health care support. These changing priorities damaged the already weak primary health care system and worsened the humanitarian crisis. Such steps can actually make the problem of COVID-19 worse. For example, although children are less affected by

COVID-19, this is only the case in countries that are not facing conflict, displacement, food insecurity, or other illness outbreaks. In Yemen, there are around two million severely malnourished under-five-year-old children, and they have a 12-times higher risk of death due to infectious diseases, such as diphtheria, measles, or COVID-19, than non-malnourished children (WaSt TIG 2018).

Second, the pandemic may put an extra emphasis on hard security and statist approaches to conflict resolution. With declining budgets and resources, peace operations are likely to pare down to what is often regarded as essential (high-level political settlements and military security) and dispense with approaches that are too often seen as nice to have but inessential—notably, local community engagement and broad humanitarian assistance that seeks to put peace on a more solid social footing for the long term. The new stripped-down policies may benefit incumbent governments at the expense of opposition groups or civil society. With cash-strapped international actors looking to find the shortest paths to stability, they may focus on shoring up the incumbent regime as the best bet. This kind of policy, searching for expediency, would reduce even further the relationships with local communities that have already suffered by COVID-19 movement restrictions.

Finally, the response to COVID-19 has made matters worse for those who are forcibly displaced by conflict. People fleeing conflict, violence, and other humanitarian disasters often face crowded camps in unsanitary conditions, discrimination, and poor access to health care, as along the United States' southern border. In the wake of COVID-19, travel restrictions and border closures have locked many into these conditions. Both COVID-19 and measures put in place to limit it have exacerbated the human toll of war.

Managing Conflict in a Post-Pandemic World

How should the world face up to conflict and violence after the pandemic and with an eye to the possibility of future pandemics? The most fundamental problems are about resources and mistrust. Investing in conflict early warning, preventive diplomacy, and peacekeeping ought to be high priorities because of how much more complex treating a pandemic becomes with war and human displacement. The same goes for fighting global food insecurity and domestic abuse. These policies are favoured both by long-run self-interest (to avoid international instability and to help stamp out a disease that is a common threat), and by sheer humanitarianism. But with the pandemic, the disruption of global supply chains, the war in Ukraine, a crisis of food insecurity and in the context of climate change, every country in the world is facing considerable economic disruption, making it hard to look outside one's own borders. Every state's pandemic response force should include a global component, with aid agencies and ministries of foreign affairs involved in decision-making in order to keep global affairs on the agenda. And, because conflicts generate refugees, states must be willing to open their borders to asylum-seekers.

International mistrust, however, makes it harder to avoid international conflict and harder to prevent and respond to civil wars. Though the virus has mainly harmed global cooperation, it also presented one paramount opportunity to restart it. Effectively collaborating on the production and distribution of a COVID-19 vaccine was critical for global public health, of course. It could have provided positive spillover effects, demonstrating that the world could take effective action to solve a pressing global crisis. The limited efforts in this regard, with the COVID-19 Vaccines Global Access (COVAX) program falling well short of its goals due to vaccine nationalism, has instead fostered disillusionment with existing institutions and with Western leadership. Over the longer term, *restoring the influence of WHO* is not just a global public health imperative but an international security imperative as well, and international security professionals should see it as such. The same goes for reestablishing the global economy.

To address the risk that international conflicts become more likely under the pandemic, it will be critical to maintain *open channels of communication*. To this end, establishing clear infectious disease protocols for conducting face-to-face diplomacy, mediation, and arms control inspections should be a priority. Much like global vaccine cooperation, diplomatic efforts should focus on the need for cooperation in the face of a common enemy. Diplomats, for example, could as a first step bracket health from other issues and focus on how pairs of rivals can help each other confront epidemics. Here, regional organizations can play an especially crucial role in assessing needs and opportunities to cooperate as part of a broader regional effort at fighting the virus and maintaining peace.

There will likely be significant mistrust to overcome in many intrastate conflict settings as well. In these settings, health authorities of all kinds should recognize that their efforts may often be met with mistrust and fear, and that this is not irrational in societies that have suffered turmoil. Government health authorities and international organizations must be willing *to cooperate with local communities and civil-society organizations*—even, in many cases, with armed opposition groups. International organizations should recognize that many of the policies that work to fight infectious disease, such as restrictions on movement, assembly, and work, are not politically neutral and are unlikely to be read as such. This is another reason to build strong dialogue between governments and opposition groups so that these policies can be designed and implemented in such a way as to reduce the potential for a backlash. Similarly, governments must be encouraged to critically evaluate their actions in the fight against COVID-19 to ensure that these do not widen gaps and do not fuel existing conflicts within societies.

Fighting pandemics requires adjustments for peace operations. These missions should *recognize that, even in outbreaks, infectious disease is far from the only problem that conflict-affected populations face.* They must continue strengthening local relationships and their engagement with civilians to the extent possible. They must make a point to reach out to populations who already face barriers to participating in decision-making, such as women, members of persecuted ethnic groups, and sexual minorities. Personnel in these operations should actively extend their gaze to consider what other health risks and forms of violence must be addressed. For humanitarian relief more generally, efforts to combat infectious disease outbreaks in conflict settings should run in parallel with strengthening primary health services. The indirect consequences of the pandemic should also be assessed, such as domestic violence, in collaboration with humanitarian organizations, and in a manner sensitive to the particular needs of distinct populations.

Canada ought to play its traditional middle-power role here, and an immediate investment in diplomacy can help it to do so. This will seem extravagant under record budget deficits, but the alternative may be even worse. It should lead the way in vaccine cooperation. In its diplomacy, Canada should ensure the inclusion of human security and gender-sensitive language in statements on pandemics and *attempt to incite and persuade governments and institutions to maintain and expand the rights of ethnic, gender, and sexual minorities.* Its aid grants, diplomatic missions, and peace operations should prioritize inclusion, trust, and a recognition of the many challenges beyond COVID-19 that exist. Canada can play a leading role in global health security response, both in convincing the world of the need for a sustained effort, and in helping to channel that effort to the needs of the most vulnerable.

References

Azcona, Ginette, Antra Bhatt, Jessamyn Encarnacion, Juncal Plazaola-Castaño, Papa Seck, Silke Staab, and Laura Turquet. 2020. *From Insight to Action: Gender Equality in the Wake of COVID-19*. New York: United Nations Entity for Gender Equality and the Empowerment of Women (UN Women). https://www.unwomen.org/en/digital-library/publications/2020/09/gender-equality-in-the-wake-of-covid-19.

Brubaker, Rebecca, and Dirk Druet. 2020. *Back from the Brink: A Comparative Study of UN Preventive Diplomacy in West and Central Africa*. New York: United Nations University.

De Coning, Cedric. 2020. "Examining the Longer-Term Effects of COVID-19 on UN Peacekeeping Operations." *The Global Observatory*, May 13, 2020. https://theglobalobservatory.org/2020/05/examining-longer-term-effects-covid-19-un-peacekeeping-operations/.

Di Razza, Namie, and Jake Sherman. 2020. *Integrating Human Rights into the Operational Readiness of UN Peacekeepers*. New York: International Peace Institute. https://www.ipinst.org/wp-content/uploads/2020/04/2004_Integrating-Human-Rights.pdf.

Ero, Comfort. 2021. "Africa's Peace and Security: The Pressures of COVID-19." Address to Off-the-Record on April 14, 2021. https://www.crisis-group.org/africa/africas-peace-and-security-pressures-covid-19.

Geneva Declaration Secretariat. 2015. *Global Burden of Armed Violence 2015: Every Body Counts*. Cambridge: Cambridge University Press.

Goldstein, Joshua S. 2011. *Winning the War on War: The Decline of Armed Conflict Worldwide*. New York: Penguin.

Harsch, Michael F., Tyler Y. Headley, and Alexandra Novosseloff. 2020. "Peacekeeping during Pandemics: How the UN Can Be Part of the Solution." *The Global Observatory*, June 3, 2020. https://theglobalobservatory.org/2020/06/peacekeeping-during-pandemics-how-un-can-be-part-of-solution/.

International Crisis Group. 2020a. "Global Ceasefire Call Deserves UN Security Council's Full Support." April 9, 2020. https://www.crisisgroup.org/global/global-ceasefire-call-deserves-un-security-councils-full-support.

———. 2020b. "Conflict, Health Cooperation and COVID-19 in Myanmar." Asia Briefing 161. Brussels: International Crisis Group. May 19, 2020. https://www.crisisgroup.org/asia/south-east-asia/myanmar/b161-conflict-health-cooperation-and-covid-19-myanmar.

Liechtenstein, Stephanie. 2020. "How COVID-19 Has Transformed Multilateral Diplomacy." *World Politics Review*, June 1, 2020. https://www.worldpoliticsreview.com/articles/28801/how-covid-19-has-transformed-multilateral-diplomacy.

Mittal, Vikram. 2022. "The Impact of the COVID-19 Pandemic on Russian Operations in Ukraine." *Forbes*, March17, 2022. https://www.forbes.com/sites/vikrammittal/2022/03/17/covid-19s-role-in-the-russian-lack-of-success-in-ukraine/?sh=113a2e9e7be2.

OCHA (United Nations Office for the Coordination of Humanitarian Affairs). 2020. *Global Humanitarian Response Plan COVID-19. United Nations Coordinated Appeal April-December 2020*. New York: OCHA. https://www.unocha.org/sites/unocha/files/Global-Humanitarian-Response-Plan-COVID-19.pdf.

Pavlik, Melissa. 2020. "A Great and Sudden Change: The Political Violence Landscape before and after the COVID-19 Pandemic." Armed Conflict Location and Event Data Project. August 4, 2020. https://acleddata.com/2020/08/04/a-great-and-sudden-change-the-global-political-violence-landscape-before-and-after-the-covid-19-pandemic/.

Pettersson, Thérése, Stina Högbladh, and Magnus Öberg. 2019. "Organized Violence, 1989–2018 and Peace Agreements." *Journal of Peace Research* 56, no. 4 (July): 589–603. https://doi.org/10.1177/0022343319856046.

Posen, Barry. 2020. "Do Pandemics Promote Peace? Why Sickness Slows the March to War." *Foreign Affairs*, April 23, 2020. https://www.foreignaffairs.com/articles/china/2020-04-23/do-pandemics-promote-peace.

Rozen, Laura. 2020. "Coronavirus Spurs Regional Humanitarian Outreach to Iran." *Al-Monitor*, March 18, 2020. https://www.al-monitor.com/pulse/originals/2020/03/coronavirus-spur-humanitarian-outreach-iran.html.

UNHCR (United Nations High Commissioner for Refugees). 2019. *Global Trends: Forced Displacement in 2019*. Geneva: UNHCR. https://www.unhcr.org/5ee200e37.pdf.

Walter, Barbara F. 2017. "The New New Civil Wars." *Annual Review of Political Science*, 20:469–486. https://doi.org/10.1146/annurev-polisci-060415-093921.

WaSt TIG (Wasting-Stunting Technical Interest Group ENN) 2018. *Child Wasting and Stunting: Time to Overcome the Separation. A Briefing Note for Policy Makers and Programme Implementers*. Oxfordshire: Emergency Nutrition Network. https://www.ennonline.net/attachments/2912/WaSt-policy-brief.pdf.

World Food Programme. 2020. *COVID-19 External Situation Report #14*. Rome: World Food Programme. https://docs.wfp.org/api/documents/14feab1255a246deb2724cf6f408504b/download?_ga=2.264801159.946802653.1599589073-2059417347.1599589073.

CHAPTER 7

Canada-U.S. Relations

Daniel Béland, Philippe Fournier,
François Furstenberg, and Pierre Martin

A s COVID-19 spread across the world, it ruthlessly exposed underlying social and institutional dysfunctions. The pandemic exploited socio-economic inequalities, ambushed creaking health and education systems, devastated eldercare facilities, and brought the world's most advanced economies to their knees. The crisis also highlighted and accelerated long-term trends in international relations. Although Canada and the United States pride themselves on a long and friendly partnership, the pandemic revealed a deep well of fragility lying just beneath the surface of cooperation and stability. Even as they remained close allies and trading partners, the two countries sharply diverged in their response to the crisis. Those divergences exposed deep-seated trends like the extreme inequality in the United States and highlighted the gradual decline of its hegemony from its mid twentieth-century peak.

When the COVID-19 pandemic hit the United States with its full force in March 2020, the uneven effects immediately manifested themselves. The American Black community and American Latin community, as well as immigrants of colour were affected at far higher rates than the white community. In the Corona neighbourhood of Queens, largely Spanish speaking and populated by immigrants both documented and not, thousands fell ill, and hundreds died; meanwhile, the wealthy enclaves of Manhattan saw an exodus of residents taking shelter in their country houses. The divergent death toll was only one facet of the structural racism that continues to shape life in the United States. Another facet was dramatically brought to the world's attention when a Minneapolis police officer murdered George Floyd in May 2020, just as the nation was emerging from lockdown. These twin crises in public health and race relations were embedded in durable forms of inequality. In this chapter, we explore these forms of inequality, as they negatively affected the international image of the United States while forcing Canadians to look at their own society and policies in the mirror of the United States. Then, we analyze the crisis of U.S. leadership associated with the Trump presidency while stressing its likely consequences on Canada-U.S. relations. We also discuss the shifts in public policy stemming from the 2020 U.S. elections, and the early months of the Biden administration, which, though it departed from the Trump administration in significant ways, found itself in the position of responding to the health, economic, and racial turmoil that had built up over the previous 40 years. This chapter ends with proposals to address the challenges of the post-COVID-19 world in North America.

Canada-U.S. Relations and the Trump Presidency

To set recent trends in historical context, it is worth taking a few steps back. In her classic 1970 book, *Silent Surrender*, the economist Kari Levitt painted a portrait of Canada's slide "into a position of economic, political, and cultural dependence on the United States" (Levitt 1970, xlv). Writing at the peak of global decolonization, Levitt traced the recolonization of Canada into a "branch-plant economy" lacking essential features of economic and political sovereignty. With its national autonomy hollowed out by a "new mercantilism" led by U.S.-based multinational corporations, Canada was in the position of supplicant, "begging favours from the metropolitan power." "Evidently," she tartly concluded, "there is a price to be paid for the special relationship" (Levitt 1970, 5).

In retrospect, Levitt's book appears as a statement of extraordinary prescience, previewing what would later be called the neoliberal global order. The past half-century has seen the ever-growing integration of the North American and global economies, particularly accelerating in the wake of the North American Free Trade Agreement (NAFTA). With a few bumps along the way, the future Levitt foresaw in 1970 has largely come to pass.

The forces that Levitt believed were dismantling Canadian sovereignty have also, perhaps ironically, hollowed out U.S. political and economic sovereignty as well. With technological innovation and the offshoring of vast amounts of U.S. manufacturing capacity, U.S. workers saw their standards of living stagnate and then decline. These forces, among others, have destabilized the U.S. political system, resulting in increasing political polarization. The first casualty of that polarization was the Republican Party, whose long-simmering current of xenophobia, racial acrimony, anti-intellectualism, and hollow conservative dogmatism culminated in the 2016 nomination of Donald Trump to the presidential ticket. The second casualty was the country itself, especially its social and political cohesion, when Trump ascended to the presidency.

It is no coincidence that the states of the old industrial core of the country tipped the balance for Donald Trump, with Ohio, Michigan, Wisconsin, and Pennsylvania shifting from Democratic blue to Republican red in 2016. Those were the areas most affected by the process of deindustrialization that had transpired in recent decades, as working-class white families saw their standards of living decline substantially. It is also the region most intimately connected to the Canadian economy, with the greatest intensity of cross-border trade.

In 2017, Donald Trump came to power vowing to remake the global economy by building a wall on the Mexican border, renegotiating NAFTA, pulling the United States out of the Trans-Pacific Partnership negotiations, and cracking down hard on trade with China. If there was any single thread to an otherwise chaotic presidency, it was this assertion of "America First" in matters of international trade and migration. Trump repeatedly pledged to "close the border" with Mexico, a commitment that seemed as impossible economically as it was powerful symbolically. His economic and foreign policies produced accelerating strains with the United States' allies and trading partners, destabilizing longstanding political and economic relations. As Trump's presidency progressed, a growing number of commentators came to predict the fracturing of the postwar, U.S.-centred global order.

It was in this context that the novel COVID-19 hit the world in the early months of 2020. Perhaps the most remarkable aspect of its power was its instantaneous and almost uncanny ability to accomplish what the Trumpian movement had so fruitlessly sought until then: to close borders and transform trade with America's foreign partners.

Inequality and the COVID-19 Crisis

In the early 1970s, burdened by high taxes and strict regulation, corporate and financial actors across the developed world launched an offensive to increase profit margins and break free of government intervention. They used their considerable resources to bend legislation to their will while shifting industrial production abroad. In the United States, the combined effect of advantageous fiscal policies, low union density, corporate governance, and deregulated financial markets has been immensely favourable to the very top income bracket (the 1 percent and especially the 0.1 percent) (Hacker and Pierson 2010). Even the financial crisis of 2008 did not fundamentally change the distribution of wealth (Urban Institute 2017). As Thomas Piketty, Emmanuel Saez, and Gabriel Zucman (2018) point out, the average pre-tax income of the bottom 50 percent has stagnated since 1980. Furthermore, if Black Americans have seen a rise in their median income since the 1970s, the wealth gap with white Americans remains astonishingly large (Piketty, Saez, and Zucman 2018). As of 2018, "median black household income was 61 per cent of median white household income" (Schaeffer 2020).

Over time, the depreciation or stagnation of wages and the loss of well-paid union jobs stirred resentment in the population, especially in areas most affected by globalization and deindustrialization like the Rust Belt. The perception that political, corporate, and financial elites furthered their own interests at the expense of working people was already deeply rooted in the run-up to Trump's election in November 2016. Evidence suggests that discontent with material conditions exacerbated the powerful undercurrents of racism beneath the surface of American life, including a (misguided) perception among working-class whites that minorities benefited disproportionately from public welfare programs (Gest 2016). Rising inequality and structural racism have chipped away at the American public's trust in institutions, weakened their democracy, and paved the way to a presidency with a distinct penchant for authoritarianism, economic isolationism, and xenophobia. Not only did Trump's presidency erode the United States' reputation in the world, but it also made political and economic relations with Canada more complicated and tense.

More generally, the fact that the world's foremost economic power has entrenched a system that rewards highly mobile financial and corporate elite has made it much harder for other countries, including Canada, to opt for higher taxes on corporations and wealthy individuals, greater investments in infrastructure and social programs, and tighter regulations on the financial sector. Ultimately, any significant reordering of the world economy along greener and more social-democratic lines will be difficult if not impossible if the United States refuses to move along.

To be sure, Canada has experienced some of the same patterns as the United States; it has just done so with less intensity. In the last 30 to 40 years, the richest Canadians have taken a greater share of national income, although income inequality has somewhat receded in the last decade (Lemieux and Riddell 2017). As in the United States, wealth and income inequality disproportionally affects women and minorities. However, higher union density and greater levels of government intervention have mitigated inequalities. Even as gross domestic product (GDP) per capita is higher in the United States, Canadian households in the bottom 56 percent of the income distribution are better off than American households in the same category; they also have access to better government benefits and more affordable health care and education (Lapointe 2019). As in the United States, racism is deeply entrenched in Canadian society and its institutions. Although Canadians like to draw favourable comparisons with their neighbours to the south, the history of settler colonialism and Indigenous dispossession lies at the heart of the Canadian experience too. Meanwhile, anti-Black racism continues to pervade policing and other governmental agencies in Canada.

Health Care and Social Policy Responses

The U.S. health care system has been the object of ferocious disagreements between Republicans and Democrats. With per capita costs far exceeding those of any other country, it is a Byzantine mix of employer and government insurance plans, state and federal guidelines, and private and public provisions. Although Barack Obama's signature legislation, the Affordable Care Act (ACA), extended coverage to 20 million Americans, 27 million remain uninsured. Donald Trump came to office promising to repeal the ACA and failed to do so by a single vote in a dramatic 2017 Senate decision. Republicans nonetheless managed to remove the federal individual mandate provision, which required nearly all U.S. citizens to purchase health insurance or face penalties. Starting in 2021, however, states like Massachusetts,

New Jersey, California, Rhode Island, and the District of Columbia imposed fines for being uninsured.

The COVID-19 crisis exposed the unique vulnerabilities and inequities of the U.S. health care system (Dorn, Cooney, and Sabin 2020). Notwithstanding its extraordinary concentration of bio-tech research, the United States proved woefully ill-prepared for the pandemic and cruelly lacked the resources (hospital beds, personnel, respirators, masks, tests, etc.) to respond adequately. The pandemic hit minorities and poor people particularly hard. Black Americans were disproportionally affected because they were more likely to work in low wage essential services jobs, to suffer from underlying health conditions, and to have less access to health care (Bouie 2020). Since health coverage for working people is mostly provided by employers, many of the Americans who lost their job during the pandemic also lost their health insurance.

Overall, the Canadian health system proved more resilient in this crisis, which suggests that universal health care coverage is a major asset in times of pandemic. Nevertheless, the pandemic high-lighted several significant weaknesses in Canadian social policy and institutions. As in the United States, it hit low-income and minority populations particularly hard, with certain groups facing higher rates of infection and unemployment. In addition, Canada's long-term care facilities proved exceptionally vulnerable to COVID-19, with death tolls in Quebec facilities reaching shocking levels.

In the realm of social and economic policy, the pandemic forced both the United States and Canada to adopt emergency measures to support businesses, the unemployed, and students. The federal government in Canada adopted bolder measures much faster than its U.S. counterpart, which faced political obstacles related to both checks-and-balances and high levels of partisan disagreement. Significantly, the more centralized approach to unemployment relief in Canada made its response more rapid and effective (Béland et al. 2021). The fragmented nature of unemployment benefits in the United States slowed the provision of emergency funds to laid-off workers. Many states saw their creaky system break down in the face of the sudden number of applications.

The United States and Canada at a Crossroads

In the United States, deep inequalities, galloping health costs, systemic racism, and environmental degradation, among other issues, have created deep-seated resentments and divisions, which have led Americans to a "declining trust in government and each other" (Rainie and Perrin 2019). Americans do not agree on the issues they confront, and still less on how to respond. Few, however, disagree that more tension and social strife would further harm the country. A younger generation has expressed its dismay at racism and inequality. It has also cast doubt on the deeply entrenched tradition of individual liberty and limited government. Perhaps the United States is in the process of turning inward as it braces for major structural changes.

Canada must also reflect on its own challenges, which include growing inequality and pervasive racial discrimination against Indigenous Peoples, Black Canadians, and other minorities. In Canada, even if COVID-19 partially and temporarily shifted focus away from this issue, the situation of Indigenous Peoples drew more national attention than in the United States, in part because of their greater demographic and political weight. While that growing attention is a positive development, it cannot hide centuries of injustices and blatant, ongoing forms of socio-economic inequality. Simultaneously, Canada must cope with a changing international context in which U.S. leadership appears to be waning.

A Lack of Domestic and International Leadership

Confronted with previous global crises, the United States often took the mantle of international leadership, as was the case in the global response to the 2008 financial crisis and, more recently, during the 2014 Ebola crisis. Not this time. Under President Trump, the United States abdicated its leading role in international institutions, and largely failed to lead by example. It mostly provided a vivid model of what *not* to do. The COVID-19 pandemic took momentous proportions in the United States mainly because it encountered a dysfunctional political system and a profoundly divided society.

Political and Institutional Dysfunctions

In January 2020, President Trump ignored multiple warnings from his intelligence services about the unusual ease of transmission and the high rates of mortality documented in China. Although there is evidence that he was informed of the acute nature of the public health threat (Woodward 2020), the president then spent much of the month of February downplaying the gravity of the situation in hope of appeasing financial markets. By the time the Trump administration finally acted, in early March, community transmission in several major metropolitan areas was already rampant. A Columbia University study released in May 2020 showed that implementing social distancing and other measures one or two weeks earlier might have saved more than 36,000 lives in the United States (Pei, Kandula, and Shaman 2020).

From March to May, a COVID-19 task force took the lead in coordinating the federal government's response and its crisis communication strategy. Unfortunately, government experts were ignored or overruled. The president's willful ignorance of scientific advice and disdain for expertise had all the hallmarks of an authoritarian regime. Suspicious of the "loyalty" of professional experts inherited from the previous administration, he chose—early in the crisis—to entrust a good part of the responsibilities for planning the pandemic strategy to his son-in-law, Jared Kushner, a policy novice with no relevant training or experience.

President Trump was motivated by his desire to see a rapid return of economic activity in the third quarter of 2020, in time for the election. He encouraged states to end their confinement measures as soon as possible. This premature reopening caused an early "second wave" in parts of the country that had been relatively spared in the early months, such as Texas, Florida, and other states in the South and West. In the long run, these late starters—nearly all governed by Republicans—managed to cumulate some of the worst records of infections, hospitalizations, and deaths, due largely to politically motivated resistance to public health recommendations. Interestingly, in Canada a similar pattern emerged in the Conservative-ruled province of Alberta, which was initially spared from the worst effects of the pandemic, and where political resistance to mitigation measures contributed to make the later stages of the crisis dramatically worse.

Political polarization lurked behind the precipitous reopening. A growing ideological, political, and even epistemological gap between Democrats and Republicans reached a peak during the Trump presidency. Democrats and Republicans struggled to find common ground on basic policy issues, a situation that exacerbated legislative stalemate after Democrats regained control of the House of Representatives after the 2018 midterms. In some cases, the consequences were obvious, as when the president threatened to cut federal aid to the states most affected by the first wave of infections because they were governed by Democrats. Even more damagingly, political polarization made it difficult to engage the entire population in strategies such as social distancing and mask wearing to limit the spread of the virus. Throughout 2020, in the United States, polls showed vast differences between Democrats and Republicans in perceptions of the risk and of measures to minimize it.

A Politicized and Weakened Administrative State

A major reason the federal government found itself so unprepared for COVID-19 was President Trump's decision to dismantle a global health security unit put in place by the previous administration to coordinate pandemic response. The resulting bureaucratic disorganization led, notably, to an inefficient distribution of key supplies, such as ventilators or personal protective equipment for hospital use. The lack of coordination impeded a coherent strategy of testing and contact tracing, which accelerated the propagation of the virus. Even as the number of tests increased markedly through the summer, the capacity to produce timely results and provide adequate contact tracing was sorely lacking.

Another striking example of the Trump administration's assault on essential administrative infrastructures during the initial phases of the COVID-19 crisis came when the White House fired the Department of Health and Human Services' Inspector General, Christi Grimm, as she was homing in on the department's lack of preparedness for, and mishandling of, the pandemic response.

Despite the relative success of the Trump White House in its push for speedy vaccine development and testing, dubbed "Operation Warp Speed," the Republican leadership had no unified plan for an effective nationwide distribution of the vaccines, which was left almost entirely to states, and withheld crucial data from the Biden transition team. Consequently, the incoming Biden administration had to build its own plan from scratch.

Overall, in the context of the early responses to the pandemic, the Trump administration weakened the capacity of the U.S. federal government to address global health crises, a situation that created direct and negative implications for Canada, which shares such a long border with the United States.

A Deficit of International Leadership

Whether U.S. international leadership is conceived as structural predominance, hegemony, or merely the pretension to stand as a model for others to emulate, as the Founders envisioned, the initial responses to the COVID-19 crisis marked a low point in—some might venture to say the end of—U.S. leadership.

Such assertions should be made with care. U.S. hegemonic decline has been announced for decades, and yet the United States had repeatedly managed to re-establish its predominance. After the crises of the 1970s and the ensuing predictions of the end of hegemony, the United States retained its role as the indispensable power, particularly in the early years after the fall of communism in the former Soviet Union and Eastern Europe. While its interventions in the crises that followed the Cold War were not uniformly commendable, successive administrations expressed a willingness to use U.S. power to serve global economic interests such as free trade that many considered essential to their own national interests. U.S. dominance has been notably clear in international finance. In close collaboration with the International Monetary Fund, the U.S. Treasury has been involved in various episodes of "failure containment" after major financial crises since the 1980s, most notably in Latin America and East Asia (Gindin and Panitch 2013).

In some instances, the will to global leadership probably did more harm than good, as in the invasion of Iraq. One can argue that the global recession of 2008 was a direct consequence of inherent weaknesses and abuses in the U.S. financial system. Yet, when it came time to spearhead a coordinated international response to the recession, U.S. leadership asserted itself (Drezner 2014). The chaotic withdrawal from Afghanistan in 2021 put the limits of U.S. foreign policy into sharp focus. The 20-year drive towards nation building and democracy promotion largely failed. Whilst the United

States invested the bulk of its resources into building up the security apparatus in Afghanistan, it enabled corrupt and incompetent leadership and failed to foster political legitimacy, order, or security. The hasty and poorly planned withdrawal also rattled U.S. allies who took part in successive NATO missions. The United States' decision has cast doubt on the long-term viability of the alliance. The episode showed that the strains that developed in the alliance during the Trump years did not entirely disappear when Joe Biden assumed the presidency. It also confirmed the pivot towards geopolitical competition with China. Ironically, China might be the prime beneficiary of U.S. retreat in the region.

Although U.S. hegemony in the Obama years encountered its share of setbacks (e.g., the muddled intervention in Libya and Russia's increased influence over Syria and the Middle East more generally), U.S. leaders broadly maintained their commitment to multilateral forums on matters of security, economic affairs, and the environment. In all these areas, the arrival of Donald Trump in the White House back in January 2017 marked a sharp turn from multilateral engagement, and it might take several years for subsequent administrations to replenish the country's reservoir of good will among international allies and partners.

Examples of this pattern include the country's withdrawal from the Trans-Pacific Partnership and its efforts to transform the United Nations Security Council into a forum for global strategic competition between the United States and China. Although COVID-19 combined the greatest public health crisis with the deepest economic recession since the Second World War, the Trump administration used the opportunity to announce its intention to withdraw from the World Health Organization (WHO). This move, part of a broader pattern of disengagement, came at a critical time for the organization tasked with coordinating international efforts to combat a global pandemic. To add fuel to the fire, President Trump exacerbated international tensions and weakened potential global coordination by regularly emphasizing competition rather than collaboration in medical research and public policy while using divisive and racist terms such as "Wuhan virus."

To fill the void left by this abdication of leadership, China made efforts to increase its presence in the relevant international forums while offering material help to individual countries. Much of the dismal state of U.S. international leadership throughout the COVID-19 crisis stemmed from the personality of the president, Donald Trump and the movement he inspired, which is likely to remain a major force in U.S. politics in the foreseeable future. There is no guarantee that his successors will be able to rebuild what has been lost as the task of confronting a global pandemic eventually gives way to that of reconstructing a badly damaged global economy.

What does this waning U.S. leadership mean for Canada-U.S. relations? Most immediately, the Trump administration forced upon Canada and Mexico a difficult renegotiation of the North American Free Trade Agreement (NAFTA) resulting in the newly labelled agreement, the Canada-United States-Mexico Agreement (CUSMA). Lest any observer see that new treaty as a renewed commitment to transborder partnership, the United States almost immediately followed its implementation by imposing new aluminum tariffs on Canada. The lesson for Canada could hardly have been clearer: its largest trading partner can no longer be a reliable ally. At the very best, the relationship is subject to the contingencies of political leadership. Canada was not the only recipient of fickle U.S. dynamics. Trump damaged historic relations with many of the United States' key allies, reorienting U.S. relations towards autocratic states such as Saudi Arabia and Russia, and away from traditional partners like Canada, France, or Germany. This reorientation will inevitably shuffle Canada's strategic alliances, hopefully towards stronger engagement with the European Union and other international partners. Most generally, however, the weakening of essential multilateral institutions damages Canada's ability to exert its influence on the world stage, insofar as those institutions have often served as the vehicle for Canadian action abroad.

Rebuilding after the Storm

President Biden has confronted the myriad challenges emerging from the pandemic and its economic fallout, compounded by the challenge of rebuilding trust in political institutions after President Trump. Donald Trump left the White House, just barely, but the political climate that his one-term presidency created is not about to dissipate. Indeed, the assault on the U.S. Capitol during the counting of the electoral ballots signalled the difficulties of polarization, rapid demographic change, racial tensions, culture wars, a corrosive media environment, growing inequalities, and the frustration of all those stuck in the waiting line for the American dream.

The aftermath of the pandemic and of the wave of unrest in 2020 and 2021 will further complicate the task of rebuilding. The pandemic left behind an economy in tatters and public finances saddled with much higher levels of public debt. Total public debt climbed from 87 percent of GDP in 2019 to 118 percent in 2020 in Canada. In the United States, public debt grew from 108 percent of GDP to a staggering 127 percent in the same period (IMF 2021). This public debt may prove to be an economic drag if interest rates return to substantially higher levels. More generally, reconstruction will take time and political will.

During the first months of the Biden administration, Congress enacted massive stimulus measures, unleashing a debate about which, if any, to make permanent. The Child Tax Credit, for example, has the clear potential to dramatically reduce child poverty in the United States. And yet its retention is far from assured. This type of measure, which has led commentators to label Biden as a "crusader for the poor," could have a long-term impact on social policy and economic inequality in the United States. Beyond Biden, the attention to poverty and inequality reduction in the United States is a sign of the growing influence of the progressive wing of the Democratic Party, a situation facilitated by the Democratic control of Congress in the aftermath of the 2020 federal elections (Béland et al. 2022). However, as we have seen with the Social Spending Bill, disagreements between centrists and progressives in both houses of Congress could lead to protracted struggles over the size and scope of Biden's proposed reforms.

Beyond social policy, the Biden administration has embraced a pro-science approach that facilitates the fight against COVID-19. Yet vaccination rates in the United States are now lower than in Canada, a situation related in part to a higher level of vaccine hesitancy—or outright resistance—in "red states." These internal ideological and political divisions are also felt in the disparities among states in the ongoing public health responses to the pandemic.

Simultaneously, the factors that led to Trump's rise, such as xenophobia, isolationism, protectionism, and his zero-sum view of the world—when other countries do well the United States must be losing—remain in the political environment. Even under the Biden administration, these forces remain obstacles to a return to the liberal internationalism that formed the ideological underpinning of U.S. leadership for several decades, and by implication to Canada's ability to exert its own influence. Regaining the trust of key allies, especially in Europe, will take years. Until and unless some form of bipartisan consensus on the fundamental tenets of U.S. international engagement is restored, U.S. leadership will remain impaired, with Canada largely adrift until it establishes a new vision for itself in the world.

Canada-U.S. Relations after the Pandemic

Although Canada fared better than the United States in the fight against COVID-19, its economy cannot fully recover until the U.S. economy does. When it comes to public health, the economy and, to some extent, politics, we are all in the same boat. As long as the United States remains Canada's dominant neighbour and largest trading partner, some degree of dependence on its political and economic health is inevitable.

As was the case in the aftermath of the tragic events of 11 September 2001, the slow reopening of land borders between the two countries as the pandemic receded may be a sign that the goal of unfettered economic integration between the two countries faces enormous political obstacles and will remain elusive.

Although small U.S. towns and businesses near the Canadian border and tourism were most impacted by the exceptionally long and symbolically charged closure of the border for non-essential reasons, trade between the two countries remained strong. However, reopening the border presented various logistical and political challenges, which hampered the fluidity of cross-border exchanges for some time.

Beyond it, Canadian public health officials will need to cooperate with their U.S. counterparts to manage possible new outbreaks of the virus—and of other diseases. There will be much to learn from the shared experiences of COVID-19 outbreaks in long-term care facilities, where a huge number of COVID-19 infections and deaths point to urgent policy changes regarding the health care of older adults in both countries. Located below the radar screen of partisan politics, this form of policy learning should involve the states and the provinces, which are at the centre of the public health fight against the pandemic on the ground.

Although most jobs lost during the pandemic were not related to trade, Canada's export-dependent sectors are likely to recover slowly from the shock that ensued. They will continue to suffer until demand levels in the United States recover and will also be threatened by the possibility of new barriers to trade and to trans-border production chains. There is no *a priori* reason to expect long-term prohibitive obstacles to the flow of goods across the Canada-U.S. border once the proper measures are in place to mitigate the risks. The experience of bilateral trade in the wake of the 11 September 2001 attacks and the border controls that were subsequently put in place shows that their impact on bilateral can be minimized, something that Canada did in 2001–2002 by showing leadership regarding this important file. The impact on tourism and in-person services trade, however, is likely to be substantial and potentially long-lasting.

More broadly, Canada has much to learn from the rocky political experiences of the United States during the pandemic. From the point of view of crisis management, the U.S. example has shown the deadly consequences of mixed messages and the politicization of public health directives. There will also be lessons from the U.S. experience concerning the workings of federalism. In particular, the U.S. case revealed the dangers of competition between states and between levels of government in a public health crisis. Canada more successfully tackled this issue than the United States thanks to better intergovernmental coordination and more limited partisan interference. Finally, just as the U.S. experience with COVID-19 shows the deadly effects of income and racial inequalities, it has also highlighted the risks posed by the combination of prejudice and incompetence in political leadership at the state, local, and national levels.

Ironically, the Canada-U.S. border, which was a key source of anxiety in the United States after the attack on 11 September 2001, became a major source of anxiety in Canada, regarding both COVID-19 and migration. Time will tell whether this negative Canadian perception of the Canada-U.S. border will endure beyond the COVID-19 pandemic.

Ideas to Improve the North American Afterworld

From the perspective of Canada-U.S. relations, considering the impacts of growing inequality and leadership challenges discussed above, what ideas should we promote for the post-pandemic world? This final section emphasizes the need for concrete collaboration among non-governmental, civil society organizations from both sides of the Canada-U.S. border. This perspective is grounded in the assumption that Canada-U.S. relations cannot be reduced to governmental actors and that, when government fails, as is the case in the United States during the Trump presidency, it is appropriate to improve international ties by going above and beyond formal institutional "veto players" in that country. With this in mind, we have four main suggestions about how to improve the North American Afterworld.

First, as social scientists, we must remain aware that our ability to predict the future is inherently limited, especially in times of acute global uncertainty. Consequently, the first thing to do is to *closely monitor the situation* and, in the case of Canada's relationship with the United States, take a systematic look at how the COVID-19 policy situation evolves at both the federal and the state levels. This includes the subnational level, where states continue to act as "laboratories of democracy." Here, more regular interactions between Canadian and U.S. subnational (provincial and state) officials about the best policy practices on the ground in terms of both public health and social policy, could help improve responses to the pandemic on both sides of the border.

Second, we can *draw political and policy lessons from the differences between Canada and the United States* in the handling of the COVID-19 crisis. For instance, the level of partisan and inter-governmental conflict appeared stronger on average in the United States than in Canada, where a consensus over the serious nature of the public health emergency crystallized rapidly, as evidenced by polling data (Merkley et al. 2020). Yet, partisan divergence in perceptions of government responses exists on both sides of the border, which suggests we should not exaggerate the gap between the two countries, as far as public opinion is concerned. This cautionary remark cannot hide the fact that intergovernmental conflict during the first months of the COVID-19 crisis was lower in Canada than in the United States. Systematic research about the causes and consequences of these differences in intergovernmental patterns would be helpful to *improve intergovernmental governance in both countries* in the wake of the COVID-19 pandemic.

Beyond political parties and the workings of federalism, a comparison between how Canada and the United States fared during the COVID-19 crisis could help us better grasp the interaction between socio-economic inequalities and public health outcomes. Crucial issues here include gender and ethno-racial inequalities, as they relate not only to economic cleavages but differential access to health care, an issue particularly crucial in the United States, a country without universal coverage. Comparing the responses and impacts of

COVID-19 in Canada and the United States will help us understand the potential intersections between these inequalities and the nature of the safety net available in each country and in each state/province/territory within. This type of comparative Canada-U.S. research could help policy makers in each country identify lessons from policy successes and failures with the hope of *improving health and social programs* where needed.

Third, beyond the need for a more coordinated approach between state and economic actors in both countries, civil society organizations also have a key role to play in crafting the future. Unions, non-governmental organizations, and social movements have linked up for decades in the North American space. Although convergence is more tangible whenever the United States and Canada negotiate trade agreements, *civil society groups* in both countries must strive to *create institutions and mechanisms* that reflect shared democratic aspirations on human rights (including measures on racial discrimination), labour rights, and climate change. A more progressive and holistic bilateral relationship rests on the will of a public constituency, and not solely on high-level bureaucrats, politicians, and corporate and financial actors. In the current context, a growing number of citizens in both countries are calling for a fairer and greener economy. Decision makers would do well to keep these insistent demands in mind as they attempt to rebuild national economies.

Fourth, we should recall that, during the COVID-19 crisis, in large part because of the attitude of the Trump administration, the United States gave up its traditional role as the leader in global crisis management. As we look for global cooperation and solutions to the ongoing challenges Canada and the rest of the world face, we should not wait for U.S. leadership. Indeed, we may no longer be able to assume that the United States is a reliable partner in troubled times. We must develop *new strategic partnerships and increase existing relationships* with other countries to compensate for the vacuum of global U.S. leadership so apparent during the recent COVID-19 crisis. For example, Canada could play a major role in improving the capacity and the global stance of WHO, an organization that is more essential today than ever before, despite what Trump has suggested. Simultaneously, we need to keep working with the United States to properly manage the Canada-U.S. border while addressing ongoing bilateral immigration, tourism, and trade issues. In other words, the emphasis on multilateralism and non-governmental actors should not mean that high-level cooperation and dialogue between our two countries are no longer necessary.

Conclusion

As we think about rebuilding our country, Canada-U.S. relations, and the international system in the aftermath of the COVID-19 crisis and in the context of a pervasive political crisis in the United States, we should not simply strive to return to "normal." A return to the *status quo ante* is largely what happened in the aftermath of the Great Recession that followed the 2008 financial crisis. The crisis facing the world now is more dramatic and consequential than recent episodes, economically, socially, and politically. Rethinking our society and the world order requires an open mind, a willingness to develop new partnerships and allies, and the capacity to revisit old ideas like "interdependence," "protectionism," "security," and "solidarity" to face fresh challenges. This search for new ideas is especially the case when we consider the ongoing threat of climate change that, combined with the COVID-19 crisis and its socio-economic and political impacts, constitutes an existential challenge, which Canada and the rest of the world must meet with both imagination and determination.

References

Béland, Daniel, Shannon Dinan, Philip Rocco, and Alex Waddan. 2021. "Social Policy Responses to COVID-19 in Canada and the United States: Explaining Policy Variations between Two Liberal Welfare State Regimes." *Social Policy & Administration* 55, no. 2 (March): 280–294.

Béland, Daniel, Shannon Dinan, Philip Rocco, and Alex Waddan. 2022. "COVID-19, Poverty Reduction, and Partisanship in Canada and the United States." *Policy and Society* 41, no. 2 (June): 291–305.

Bouie, Jamelle. 2020. "Why Coronavirus Is Killing African-Americans More Than Others." *The New York Times*, April 14, 2020. https://www.nytimes.com/2020/04/14/opinion/sunday/coronavirus-racism-african-americans.html.

Dorn, Aaron V., Rebecca E. Cooney, and Miriam L. Sabin. 2020. "COVID-19 Exacerbating Inequalities in the US." *The Lancet* 395, no. 10232 (April): 1243–1244.

Drezner, Daniel. 2014. *The System Worked: How the World Stopped Another Great Depression*. Oxford: Oxford University Press.

Gest, Justin. 2016. *The New Minority: White Working Class Politics in an Age of Immigration and Inequality.* Oxford: Oxford University Press.

Gindin, Sam, and Leo Panitch. 2013. *The Making of Global Capitalism: The Political Economy of American Empire.* London and New York: Verso Books.

Hacker, Jacob S., and Paul Pierson. 2010. "Winner-Take-All Politics: Public Policy, Political Organization, and the Precipitous Rise of Top Incomes in the United States." *Politics & Society* 38, no. 2: 152–204. https://doi.org/10.1177/0032329210365042.

IMF (International Monetary Fund). 2021. "World Economic Outlook Database, International Monetary Fund (April)." https://www.imf.org/en/Publications/WEO/weo-database/2021/April.

Lapointe, Simon. 2019. *Household Incomes in Canada and the United States: Who Is Better Off?* CSLS Research Report 2019-01. Ottawa: Centre for the Study of Living Standards. http://www.csls.ca/reports/csls2019-01.pdf.

Lemieux, Thomas, and Craig W. Riddell. 2017. "Who Are Canada's Top 1 Percent?" In *Income Inequality: The Canadian Story*, edited by David A. Green, Craig W. Riddell and France St-Hilaire, 103–156. Montréal: Institute for Research on Public Policy.

Levitt, Kari. 1970. *Silent Surrender: The Multinational Corporation in Canada.* Toronto: Macmillan of Canada.

Merkley, Eric, Aengus Bridgman, Peter John Loewen, Taylor Owen, Derek Ruths, and Oleg Zhilin. 2020. "A Rare Moment of Cross-Partisan Consensus: Elite and Public Response to the COVID-19 Pandemic in Canada." *Canadian Journal of Political Science* 53, no. 2: 311–318. https://doi.org//10.1017/S0008423920000311.

Pei, Sen, Sasikiran Kandula, and Jeffrey Shaman. 2020. "Differential Effects of Intervention Timing on COVID-19 Spread in the United States." *Science Advances* 6, no. 49 (December): eabd6370. https://doi.org//10.1126/sciadv.abd6370.

Piketty, Thomas, Emmanuel Saez, and Gabriel Zucman. 2018. "Distributional National Accounts: Methods and Estimates for the United States." *The Quarterly Journal of Economics* 133, no. 2 (May): 553–609. https://doi.org/10.1093/qje/qjx043.

Rainie, Lee, and Andrew Perrin. 2019. "Key Findings about Americans' Declining Trust in Government and Each Other". New York: Pew Research Center. July 22, 2019. https://www.pewresearch.org/fact-tank/2019/07/22/key-findings-about-americans-declining-trust-in-government-and-each-other/.

Schaeffer, Katherine. 2020. "6 Facts about Economic Inequality in the U.S." New York: Pew Research Center. February 7, 2020. https://www.pewresearch.org/fact-tank/2020/02/07/6-facts-about-economic-inequality-in-the-u-s/.

Urban Institute. 2017. "Nine Charts about Wealth Inequality in America." Last modified October 5, 2017. http://apps.urban.org/features/wealth-inequality-charts/index.html.

Woodward, Bob. 2020. *Rage*. New York: Simon & Schuster.

CHAPTER 8

Human Rights

Cynthia Milton, Pearl Eliadis, Pablo Gilabert,
Frédéric Mégret, and René Provost

Our COVID-19 moment—a suspended time of unknown duration—gave us an opportunity to reflect upon what human rights mean in a global context when we are faced with an emergency that limits them. It was difficult to take to the streets because we might put ourselves and others in harm's way. Still, George Floyd's death at the hands of U.S. police propelled people from their homes to demand the end of systemic racism around the world. This outpouring tells us that the notion of rights remains salient and powerful. Yet we have also seen human rights increasingly threatened by non-democratic efforts to consolidate power and silence dissent. The tension between a strong civil society (and transnational networks) and an uncivil state and non-state actors that all vie for their notion of rights (or their suppression) makes human rights a double-edged concept in the context of the pandemic, depending on who is defining them or infusing them with meaning. While in some parts of the world, the return of the state has meant a renewed guarantor of these rights, in other parts it has meant a powerful actor is able to dismantle them.

The authors of this chapter hope to prompt a discussion of specific rights and pressure points that came to light in the time of COVID-19, and how we might address these rights and fragilities in the world after the pandemic. First, and most immediately, we discuss how governments, citizens, and the international community risk normalizing emergency measures and eroding state accountability, and thereby curtailing civil liberties. Next, we turn to two concrete examples of pressure points: the unequal rights of individuals and communities in diasporas, and the need to actively protect labour rights as human rights (in particular as social and economic rights). The concluding section offers a series of questions and calls for international solidarity around a human rights framework in our post-COVID-19 world. Rights can form the basis upon which new solidarities may be built in the aftermath of this difficult historical turning point.

The Normalization of Emergency Measures

In the early days of the COVID-19 crisis, Italian philosopher Giorgio Agamben (2020a) published a polemic that raised alarm at the breadth of restrictions imposed by his government in view of the scientific assessment of the pandemic threat in Italy at the time. While we might dispute some aspects of Agamben's argument, or the extent of his claims, the general question he raised is worth pondering: are we experiencing a tectonic shift in the overall balancing of competing values and interests that underpin the international human rights law regime? The pandemic is ongoing, but it seems a real possibility that this crisis will indeed profoundly alter, in some ways, the protection of fundamental rights and freedoms under international law.

The central concern expressed by Agamben is that the state of emergency is being erected as a new governing paradigm. He warns against the exploitation of the vagueness of the risk of contagion by political authorities to devalue all facets of life apart from biological survival, what he calls "bare life." Fear of contagion establishes every individual as a vector of threat and imposes health as a legal obligation for all. This justifies the fragmentation of communities and society at large into individuals who must socially distance or, at best, form bubbles, in ways that deny fundamental relations based on family, friendship, religion, and other constituents of individual and collective identities. In a stark rebuttal of the motto of both the French Revolutionary regime as well as the state of New Hampshire, "Live Free or Die," liberty is traded for a sense of physical safety. "It is legitimate to ask whether such a society can still be defined as human or if the loss of sensitive relationships, of face, of friendship, of love, truly can be compensated by an abstract and presumably completely illusory health security," writes Agamben (2020b) in a follow-up essay.

There is much that can be and has been criticized in Agamben's approach, including his initial denial that the pandemic posed a health risk that was more than marginal. One way to interrogate his basic claim that the health emergency normalizes a state of exception coextensive with oppression is to examine it through the lens of the human rights law regime. After all, many of the values seen as displaced or marginalized by "biosecurity" correspond to rights and freedoms protected by specific legal standards. Human rights, lest we forget, are designed for the very purpose of limiting state power, as a bulwark against the oppression that Agamben sees as incipient in current measures imposed to control the pandemic. The possibility that there may be an emergency that requires exceptional measures has been built into major human rights treaties such as the International Covenant on Civil and Political Rights, the European Convention on Human Rights, and the American Convention on Human Rights. The condition precedent for derogation under these treaties is the existence of a "threat to the life of the nation."

In a statement issued in April 2020, the UN Human Rights Committee "acknowledge[d] that States parties confronting the threat of widespread contagion may resort, on a temporary basis, to exceptional emergency powers and invoke their right of derogation from the Covenant" (2020, para. 2). The committee reminded states that, even if the pandemic can justify the suspension of fundamental rights, the measures taken must be strictly tailored to the exigencies of the situation, must not be discriminatory, and cannot justify suspending a list of rights described as "non-derogable" (never liable to suspension). It is likely that most of the measures adopted by many governments in their attempt to limit community transmission of the virus, such as restriction of movement, closing of international borders, even infringement of privacy, would be considered as necessary and proportionate by the UN Human Rights Committee or the European and Inter-American Courts of Human Rights. Derogations must be limited as to place, time, and substance to what is required to meet the public health emergency, with the overriding concern to restore full respect of protected rights and freedoms as soon as the health emergency has abated. In principle, this answers Agamben's call to return to the *status quo ante* once the pandemic has been controlled.

Despite built-in mechanisms meant to equip the human rights regime to manage emergencies rather than be displaced by them, there are nevertheless reasons to be concerned that the post-pandemic world will occasion a deeper and more systemic weakening of the protection of human rights. A first set of reasons is internal to the human rights treaty regime itself. Treaties are explicit in their regulation of derogation of rights in times of emergency, specific in their list of rights that cannot be suspended even when faced with a threat to the life of the nations, and unequivocal in asserting the power of supervisory bodies to monitor the lawfulness of derogation measures. Nevertheless, the relevant norms still leave governments a very wide discretion in deciding which restrictions to impose and for how long, referred to in Europe as the "margin of appreciation." It is not unheard of for restrictions imposed by a plurality of states in a time of crisis, like the current pandemic, to become permanent. For instance, there was a visible shift of that nature in the "global war on terror" following the attacks on 11 September 2001, with many governments that are stalwarts of the human rights regimes adopting measures that would previously have been regarded as too extreme to be justifiable. In turn, other governments that were more reluctant participants in the human rights project took advantage of what they saw to be the lowered bar for what are tolerable constraints to liberties under international law. Over time, some of these emergency measures were struck down by national courts or withdrawn by the executive, but others became permanent limits to rights and freedoms.

Another set of reasons weakening human rights protections is external to the human rights treaty regime. The derogation framework incorporated into the covenant and the European and American Conventions is not present in the African Charter of Human and Peoples' Rights, nor in other important human rights instruments like the Convention on the Rights of the Child and the Convention on the Rights of Persons with Disabilities, raising challenging questions as to how to construe the legality of emergency measures adopted under these regimes to stem the pandemic. Other states are not parties to any of these treaties, begging the question of the possibility of derogation of human rights under customary international law. Singapore, for example, is not a party to any general human rights treaty and early on used a contact tracing app that was voluntary for all, except migrant workers, who have also been subject to severe restrictions on their movements not applicable to the rest of the population; it is unclear whether the prohibition of discriminatory derogation measures found in the covenant has a parallel in customary international law (Asher 2020).

Previous systemic challenges to human rights law such as the global wave of anti-terrorism measures adopted after 2001 show that there are limits to the resilience of the human rights regime. The more profound and permanent changes have affected the most vulnerable populations, in particular migrants, who were caught in the generalized phenomenon of the securitization of migration. This time, as we see with the Singapore example, it may again be the largely disenfranchised migrant populations who suffer most acutely from newly acceptable restrictions to rights and freedoms. Other shifts tilting the accepted balance of restrictive measures and protected rights may touch upon less visible, but still tangible and immediate interests such as privacy (see chapter 4). An emergency, like this pandemic, may not be the feared gateway to oppression, but we would be deluded to deny that it may erode in a lasting and significant way international protection of human rights.

The Curtailment of Civil Liberties

COVID-19 posed a new kind of threat that looked and felt very different from military conflicts and insurgencies—the usual contexts in which human rights are most overtly challenged. With this pandemic, there were no internments of enemy aliens and spies, and no mass arrests or disappearances. Instead, people were restricted from gatherings, required to physically distance themselves and wear masks, had their mobility rights, employment, and education limited based on proof of vaccination, and were obligated to self-isolate as a result of public health edicts and sweeping emergency powers. In Canada, for instance, civil liberties historically have been treated as "core" individual rights with immediate legal effect, opposable against the state, and justiciable—meaning that one can easily go to court to protect them. Under the emergency measures, these liberties were rapidly subordinated to collective health rights—rights that had usually been seen as non-justiciable—all this without any constitutional change or legislative debate. And yet, basic freedoms such as the freedom of association and peaceful assembly have been partially suspended. Collective agreements between employers and union members have been upended and police have been given exceptional powers, including the authority to track and detain people who violate quarantine or who are believed to have gathered in violation of new rules. Between March and August 2020 alone, the Quebec and federal governments in

Canada issued 107 emergency decrees, ministerial orders, and orders-in-council related to the pandemic, including for travel and quarantine matters. Two thirds of them directly affected civil liberties. Some, notably those related to physical distancing and banning assemblies, would be likely to survive constitutional challenge. Others, like provincial bans on interprovincial travel affecting people needing to reach homes or jobs, were not. The same applies to the closing of the Canada-U.S. border, inasmuch as it blocked people whom the courts determined to be legitimate refugee claimants despite their passage through the United States to come to Canada.[1]

Emergency may allow for oppression as authorities use public health imperatives as convenient justification for actions against pro-democracy activism in Hong Kong and Black Lives Matter protests in the United States, or to avoid scrutiny and disperse public dissent for renewed oil and gas exploration and extraction in Canada; as Alberta's Energy Minister openly noted, "now is a great time [...] because you can't have protests of more than fifteen people" (Woods 2020). By invoking "biosecurity," autocrats and populist regimes on both the left and right have taken advantage of this national and international health crisis to stage "coronavirus coups." In countries such as Hungary, Brazil, and the Philippines, extraordinary measures have been deployed with no discernable connection to infection control and, rather, have been used to suppress political or popular opposition. In fragile political environments where the pandemic is compounded by conflict and multiple crises (economic, environmental, and social), the advent of COVID-19 is placing additional strain on already weak governance mechanisms, aggravating conditions for citizens' access to basic rights. In conflict environments, confinement measures have made it more difficult to uphold humanitarian law, for instance, for those housed in refugee camps.

The sweeping nature of emergency measures makes them inherently insensitive to the conditions of specific groups, including vulnerable groups and poor communities—groups that were already in crisis before the pandemic. Socio-economically disadvantaged communities have been unable to engage in social distancing or have been forced to do jobs that endanger their health. Older adults have been isolated and subjected to conditions that have sickened or killed them. Undocumented workers, workers in informal sectors, and asylum seekers have all experienced devastating consequences as borders were shut and jobs were lost with no access to public assistance.

Mobility, Diasporas, and the Coronavirus

One example of a pressure point on the human rights regime is in the realm of mobility and citizenship. As the chapter on migration and citizenship also documents, the COVID-19 pandemic has brought into stark relief that rights are experienced differently for diasporic communities. Canadian nationals abroad and foreign nationals in Canada, including dual nationals, have been affected in many specific ways by the coronavirus and the response to it. This includes health-related impediments to mobility, preventing these individuals from returning to either their country of origin or their country of residence; forms of racism and discrimination of people of Chinese or Asian ancestry, who have been the victims of racial invective based on the perceived origin of the coronavirus; special vulnerabilities in the workplace in a context where the safety of migrant workers, particularly seasonal ones, has been jeopardized.

Diasporas are a salient example that rights violations often take a complex and transnational dimension across borders, where the acts of two or several sovereign nations, coordinated or not, can impact their populations' lives. This exposes the specific vulnerabilities of those who uneasily straddle borders and the need to devise approaches that monitor their rights condition across the entire spectrum of the diasporic experience.

Diasporic communities stand to be affected in terms of their mobility rights. The pandemic has triggered a complex chain of reactions involving both border closures and efforts at repatriation. The right to family life may be impacted as family members are prevented from rejoining each other. The pandemic has shed light on the vulnerability of certain expatriates—migrant workers but also some students for example—who do not have the citizenship of their country of residence, and thus face the risk that they may be forced out or denied re-entry despite permanent residency. Some members of diasporas, particularly migrant workers, have been made to feel unwanted in several regions of the world. Even people normally accustomed to experiencing a high degree of mobility have encountered increased obstacles when travelling.

Moving back and forth between the country of origin and the country of residence is often the essence of diasporic life for economic, cultural, and personal purposes. This quality of life is fundamentally impoverished by limited and discriminatory mobility policies on many levels. Economically, the ripple effects of the pandemic will be felt for a long time to come as remittances dry out; psychologically, impediments to mobility may exact a high toll; politically, diasporas may be targeted and even scapegoated.

Some states of origin stepped up to provide support to their nationals abroad. This may include financial assistance to help the unemployed survive in their country of residence in a context where repatriation is not an option. Some states intervened forcefully on behalf of their citizens threatened by COVID-19. For example, Mexico defended Mexican migrant workers in Canada who had been infected by the coronavirus, going as far as to say it would prevent further workers from going to Canada until their security could be ensured.

Beyond this sort of assistance, initiatives at repatriation were undertaken. These efforts often fell on expatriate and migrant workers themselves. Although states of origin acted in some cases as facilitators, they also sometimes proved unable or unwilling to repatriate some of their nationals abroad. This was spectacularly the case with Australia, for example, which prevented Australians from India, then hit by the Delta variant of COVID-19, to return. The question arises as to whether there is a right to be repatriated when one cannot do so by one's own means and at least a right to return to one's country of nationality. Best practices are hard to come by, though countries such as the Philippines quite aggressively engaged in efforts to bring their nationals home. Complex issues also arose for migrant workers as a result of unpaid wages in the country of residence they often had to leave precipitously. States of nationality have a role to play in particular in pressing demands for unpaid wages in the country of residence. Efforts to not only repatriate but fully relocate returnees need to be implemented that take into account persons who may have depended on them financially.

Access to assistance and protection while abroad are powerfully mediated by forces of racialization and racism that identify the virus with certain groups, in a context where migration practices and policies had previously already taken heavily discriminatory undertones. Understanding the intersection of nationality, gender, race, and class in this context is a crucial way in which the diasporic predicament can be alleviated during a pandemic.

The Impact of COVID-19 on Labour Human Rights

Labour rights are another example of a pressure point or stress on the human rights regime, which COVID-19, as well as the national and international responses to it, has exposed and amplified. These are rights to access employment, to have decent working conditions (e.g., regarding pay, a safe and healthy work environment, and social security as a safety net), and to defend workers' interests through unionization, strikes, and other forms of associative and political action.[2] COVID-19 has negatively affected the enjoyment of these human rights in many ways including a dramatic jump in unemployment and the deterioration of work conditions. As well, COVID-19 has meant a serious rollback of workers' rights.

In Canada alone, nearly two million Canadians had lost their jobs by early May 2020, and for those that remained employed other problems came to light. While for some, working from home might have been a welcome change, for others the circumstances of working from home posed arduous challenges, such as the demand to learn new technologies swiftly, the lack of satisfactory computer equipment, and the difficulty to effectively work from a personal domicile while also homeschooling children. Other people continued to go to their regular workplace but faced serious health challenges as they did so. This was especially so for workers from disadvantaged communities. Their work sites (such as meatpacking Cargill factories or care units for older adults) were the initial hotspots for COVID-19 transmission. Their commute by public transportation also generated risks. As well, women have been disproportionally affected by labour disruption since gendered norms place a larger burden of care for dependents upon them, and women were less likely to be rehired with the opening of the economy after restrictions had been lifted.

Some firms have also curtailed their workers' right to protest against unhealthy and dangerous workplace conditions. The case of Amazon is emblematic: manual labourers in the warehouses face gruelling schedules, recurrent workplace injuries, and indignities. The right to unionization is sometimes curtailed. Salaried professionals are encouraged to scheme against each other, using an "Anytime Feedback Tool" widget to report on other workers' failures to management as they try to emerge on top at the end of each year's round of performance evaluations and layoffs (Kanto 2015; Bloodworth 2018). In the more specific context of the COVID-19 pandemic in 2020,

Amazon in the United States, after paying "almost no taxes" the previous year, offered *unpaid* time off for staff who were sick and two weeks paid leave for workers who tested positive (Kenya 2020). Employees remained obligated to complete mandatory overtime (Reich 2020).

There are several possible responses to these hardships faced by workers. First, in general, the crisis brought to the fore the important contributions of workers to our societies. When people do not work, the economy plunges, and everybody suffers. Workers are essential. The crisis is an opportunity to recognize workers' contributions, and to pair this recognition with policies that grants them conditions that allow them to fully enjoy their human rights. Their labour rights must be treated seriously and as a matter of urgency (Ferreras et al. 2020).

Second, specific programs should be devised to facilitate the maintenance of workers' jobs during the crisis, to facilitate access to jobs for those who are losing them (including through governmental initiatives in which the state acknowledges its role as employer of last resort), to resource and train workers to adapt to new technologies, to monitor the health conditions under which they work, and, finally, to protect their rights to unionize and act to defend their interests.

Third, the COVID-19 moment may be the time to experiment with a universal basic income (UBI) policy. Discussions about UBI gained traction around the world in the context of COVID-19. We have seen that the enjoyment of some human rights has actually improved in several countries through cash payments and other forms of protective social policy created during the pandemic. UBI would put a floor of dignity on which working people can stand to navigate the ongoing crisis and bargain with current and potential employers with less vulnerability.[3] Although UBI is not itself a human right, it could be seen as supportive of the fulfillment of already recognized human rights.

Minimizing the Risks of "Biosecurity" and Building International Solidarity in the Face of Emergencies

On reflecting upon the points of tension the COVID-19 moment has placed on national and international human rights frameworks, several questions have emerged. These questions cut across many of the chapters of this book as they address civil and political rights, social, cultural, and economic rights—including health—and environmental freedoms for individuals and communities, for Indigenous and non-Indigenous Peoples, migrants, refugees, and citizens:

- What are the changing obligations of states, particularly the democratic state, when collective rights to health overtake individual rights without any constitutional debate or discussion?
- What protocols based on best practices should be established to provide an evidence-based approach to emergency measures, which can be evaluated during and after the emergency?
- What are the mechanisms needed at both the international and national levels to address power abuses and attacks on the rule of law during public emergencies?
- How do we ensure that those mechanisms track the increasingly transnational trajectory of rights violations?
- How do we use human rights as a progressive tool to better understand and address the new and ongoing problems of inequality?

While in some countries, such as Canada, the coronavirus may have reinforced the state as a guarantor of basic rights, for example by reasserting basic health and economic rights, in other countries the call for "biosecurity" has been used to roll back, dismantle, or violate rights. These strains on the human rights framework suggest the critical importance of putting into place safeguards that can support participation and democratic deliberation during times of emergency and minimize the risks of normalization beyond the pandemic. There are extant national and international legal tools in place to prevent abuse of rights, even in crisis conditions, but in practice, there are already significant challenges in holding relevant actors accountable because governance mechanisms and judicial institutions are weakened or already dysfunctional.

Among the ideas that have started to take root are national mechanisms to establish or strengthen human rights. For example, on 15 April 2020, Amnesty International Canada spearheaded a public statement signed by 301 organizations and individuals encouraging the *systematic tracking and monitoring of human rights gaps in government responses* and laying the groundwork for transformative human rights reforms in Canada. Similar approaches at the international level could be used to ensure that public emergencies trigger the formation of specialized advisory groups, for example, on the situations of low-income people, marginalized groups, Indigenous Peoples, and others so that monitoring can be rapidly transformed into policy-relevant and human rights-based approaches. *Governments should provide a formal, written justification for any measure that curtails protected rights and freedoms*, to establish that it is narrowly tailored to the exigencies of the situation. As well, *governments should clearly indicate which measures are intended as temporary limitations on rights and freedoms*, and include a sunset clause setting a date at which the measures will automatically lapse unless renewed. Finally, serious thought should be given to a new special procedure at the UN Human Rights Council in the *form of a working group or special rapporteur on public emergencies to develop global standards* and ensure the *integration of health and other social rights with civil liberties* and the broader spectrum of human rights. It is clear that the "rules of the game" no longer apply to states during public emergencies, and mechanisms that would consolidate, document, and prioritize international responses to a pandemic or other emergency may create a "just in time" structure that could be readily triggered when emergencies are declared.

COVID-19 has shone a bright light upon the fragilities of our national safety nets and our international human rights regime. The problems of discrimination, inequality, and poverty all existed prior to this coronavirus. They are not new: appallingly, billions of people remain too poor to enjoy their basic human rights, despite a specious narrative of extreme poverty having fallen prior to COVID-19. As Philip Alston, outgoing UN special rapporteur on poverty wrote in July 2020, "until governments take seriously the human right to an adequate standard of living, the poverty pandemic will long outlive coronavirus." Furthermore, with nearly 80 million refugees in the world, Hannah Arendt's (1973, 296) insight remains salient: "the fundamental deprivation of human rights is manifested first and above all in the deprivation of place in the world which makes opinions significant and actions effective." Some 80 percent of refugees are in countries or territories with acute food insecurity and malnutrition, not counting exposure to COVID-19 (UNHCR 2020). Add to these inequities, the failure of wealthier nations to share vaccines casts doubt on talk of COVID-19 solidarity: as former British Prime Minister Gordon Brown decried before the World Health Organization in October 2021, it is a "moral catastrophe of historic proportions" where hundreds of millions of vaccines lie unused in the West despite the hundreds of thousands of lives that could be saved elsewhere (Rigby 2021).

Conclusion

COVID-19 makes us return again to the questions of whose rights are protected and what those rights are. As with other important historical turning points—such as the French Revolution, the UN Declaration of Human Rights, and the fall of the Berlin Wall—we witness the possible expansion of rights (civil, political, *and* social rights, economic and cultural rights, *and* most recently environmental rights) as well as to whom they are applied (women, children, Indigenous Peoples, the LGBTQ+ community) and also the possible curtailment of those rights and the marginalization of groups and individuals protected by them. We have seen in the COVID-19 moment the return to an expansive discussion of economic and social rights of migrant labourers, the civil rights of people experiencing homelessness, and the political rights of non-naturalized residents. Yet, the invocation of "human rights" as justification for not wearing a mask or not to vaccinate has expanded ever more the notion into new discursive realms. All the while, the right to health, the right to movement, the right to protest, and the rights to privacy, all seem at greater risk. And the pandemic of poverty continues on. As stated in an April 2020 UN report on COVID-19, "this is not a time to neglect human rights; it is a time when, more than ever, human rights are needed to navigate this crisis in a way that will allow us, as soon as possible, to focus again on achieving equitable sustainable development and sustaining peace" (UN 2020, 3).

In the world after COVID-19, the authors of this chapter see a great need for strong international solidarity—among global citizens' movements, non-governmental organizations (NGOs), and governments—to advance and expand the human rights agenda: on labour; health; environment; economic, social, cultural, political, and civil rights; as well as rights of self-determination, rights for individuals, and for groups. By grounding the response to the COVID-19 crisis in human rights and human dignity, we will be more likely to take the challenges faced by people who are not readily "near and dear" to us seriously. A form of cosmopolitan solidarity is called for, in which we support the rights of people around the world. Thus, for example, labour human rights should be protected across international supply chains, both at home and abroad. The search and enjoyment of new medical technologies to respond to the crisis should be a matter of international cooperation, and we should share needed medical resources with people in poorer countries on terms that are not unduly onerous to them. The human rights framing of the right to mobility and return, the defence of labour rights, both discussed above, and other rights remains productive for the well-being of individuals and communities. Human rights are universal entitlements that people have because of their humanity, not in virtue of narrower, or less morally weighty features such as their social class or nationality. They are for all.

Notes

1. The Canadian Council for Refugees et al v Minister for Immigration and Minister for Public Safety, 2020 FC 770, Canada: Federal Court, available at: https://www.refworld.org/cases,CAN_FC,5f1988484.html, accessed March 10, 2021.
2. See Universal Declaration of Human Rights, Articles 23–25. International Covenant on Economic, Social and Cultural Rights, Articles 6–9. See also Pablo Gilabert, "Labor Human Rights and Human Dignity," *Philosophy & Social Criticism* 42, no. 2 (2016): 171–199.
3. See this short interview with Philippe Van Parijs, a leading philosopher, defending UBI in the current crisis: Vittorio De Filippis, "Revenu universel 'Tout le monde aurait disposé sans délai de quoi survivre,'"May 5, 2020, 8–9, https://alfresco.uclouvain.be/alfresco/service/guest/streamDownload/workspace/SpacesStore/b4b3dd43-3a70-46d2-a286-17a3b3a63db2/2020.05.05.Libé.pdf?guest=true&fbclid=IwAR2ga40myzPR_zcCqNOyNC-02s8wyaW67tUJFrM1Mopv9dhq4SRuAYvv6FI.

References

Agamben, Giorgio. 2020a. "The Invention of an Epidemic." *Quodlibet*. February 26, 2020. www.quodlibet.it/giorgio-agamben-l-invenzione-di-un-epidemia.

———. 2020b. "Biosecurity and Politics." *Quodlibet*. May 11, 2020. www.quodlibet.it/giorgio-agamben-biosicurezza.

Alston, Philip. 2020. "Covid-19 Has Revealed a Pre-existing Pandemic of Poverty That Benefits the Rich." *The Guardian*, July 11, 2020. www.theguardian.com/global-development/2020/jul/11/covid-19-has-revealed-a-pre-existing-pandemic-of-poverty-that-benefits-the-rich.

Amnesty International. 2020. "Canada: 301 Organizations, Academics and Others Urge Governments to Adopt Human Rights Oversight of COVID-19 Responses." April 15, 2020. https://amnesty.ca/human-rights-news/canada-301-organizations-academics-and-others-urge-governments-to-adopt-human-rights-oversight-of-covid-19-responses/.

Arendt, Hannah. 1973. *Origins of Totalitarianism*. Boston: Houghton Mifflin Harcourt.

Asher, Saira. 2020. "TraceTogether: Singapore Turns to Wearable Contact-Tracing Covid Tech." *BBC News*, July 5, 2020. www.bbc.com/news/technology-53146360.

Bloodworth, James. 2018. "I Worked in an Amazon Warehouse. Bernie Sanders Is Right to Target Them." *The Guardian,* September 17, 2018. https://www.theguardian.com/commentisfree/2018/sep/17/amazon-warehouse-bernie-sanders.

The Economist. 2020. "Lost in the Amazon Jungle." January 9, 2020. https://www.economist.com/business/2020/01/09/lost-in-the-amazon-jungle.

Ferreras, Isabelle, Julie Battilana, Dominique Méda, et al. 2020. "Life After COVID-19: Decommodify Work, Democratise the Workplace." *The Wire,* May 15, 2020. https://thewire.in/economy/Covid-19-crisis-3000-researchers-600-universities-op-ed.

Gilabert, Pablo. 2016. "Labor Human Rights and Human Dignity." *Philosophy & Social Criticism* 42 (2): 171–199. https://doi.org/10.1177/0191453715603092.

———. 2018. *Human Dignity and Human Rights.* Oxford: Oxford University Press.

Kanto, Jodi, and David Streitfeld. 2015. "Inside Amazon: Wrestling Big Ideas in a Bruising Workplace." *The New York Times,* August 15, 2015. https://www.nytimes.com/2015/08/16/technology/inside-amazon-wrestling-big-ideas-in-a-bruising-workplace.html.

Kenya, Evelyn. 2020. "Amazon Fires New York Worker Who Led Strike over Coronavirus Concerns." *The Guardian,* March 31, 2020. https://www.theguardian.com/us-news/2020/mar/31/amazon-strike-worker-fired-organizing-walkout-chris-smallls

Reich, Robert. 2020. "It's Morally Repulsive how Corporations Are Exploiting this Crisis. Workers Will Suffer." *The Guardian,* March 22, 2020. https://www.theguardian.com/commentisfree/2020/mar/22/large-corporations-exploiting-coronavirus-crisis.

Rigby, Jennifer. 2021. "Failure to Share Covid Jabs a 'Historic Moral Catastrophe,' Says Gordon Brown." *The Telegraph,* October 21, 2021. https://www.telegraph.co.uk/global-health/science-and-disease/failure-share-covid-jabs-historic-moral-catastrophe-says-gordon/.

Sainato, Michael. 2020. "I'm Not a Robot': Amazon Workers Condemn Unsafe, Grueling Conditions at Warehouse." *The Guardian,* February 5, 2020. https://www.theguardian.com/technology/2020/feb/05/amazon-workers-protest-unsafe-grueling-conditions-warehouse.

Thompson, Gabriel. 2013. "The Workers Who Bring You Black Friday." *The Nation,* November 26, 2013. https://www.thenation.com/article/archive/holiday-crush/.

UN (United Nations). 2020. "COVID-19 and Human Rights: We Are All in This Together." https://unsdg.un.org/resources/covid-19-and-human-rights-we-are-all-together.

UNHCR (United Nations High Commissioner for Refugees). 2020. "1 Percent of Humanity Displaced: UNHCR Global Trends Report." Press release, June 18, 2020. https://www.unhcr.org/news/press/2020/

6/5ee9db2e4/1-cent-humanity-displaced-unhcr-global-trends-report.
html.

United Nations Human Rights Committee. 2020. *Statement on Derogations from the Covenant in Connection with the COVID-19 Pandemic.* CCPR/C/128/2 Advance unedited version, April 24, 2020. www.ohchr.org/Documents/ HRBodies/CCPR/COVIDstatement.docx.

Woods, Melanie. 2020. "Greta Thunberg Calls Out Alberta Minister Who Said It's A Great Time to Build Pipelines." *Huffpost,* May 26, 2020. https:// www.huffpost.com/archive/ca/entry/greta-thunberg-alberta-energy-minister_ca_5ecd48acc5b6ad1edf567d3f.

CHAPTER 9

COVID-19 and Inequality in the Developing World

Erik Martinez Kuhonta, Dominique Caouette,
Timothy Hodges, Christian Novak, and Maïka Sondarjee,
with the collaboration of Sonia Laszlo

The globalizing and ravaging nature of COVID-19 would have appeared, on first blush, to reinforce views, such as those of journalist Thomas Friedman (2005), that "the world is flat." Organizations like the United Nations (UN) and celebrities like Madonna have voiced a similar refrain: "we're all in this together." As the pandemic swept through New York State, former governor Andrew Cuomo famously commented that "It's the great equalizer. I don't care how smart, how rich, how powerful you think you are. I don't care how young, how old." Yet, the idea that COVID-19 is a "great equalizer" is extremely problematic. Such sentiments are fundamentally misleading because they fail to take into account the deep-seated inequalities that lie at the heart of this globalizing world, and therefore the differential struggles and challenges that the peoples of the developing world confront when dealing with a pandemic.

Instead of creating an "equalizing storm," COVID-19 has laid bare how certain countries and communities are more vulnerable to the vast and devastating consequences of this pandemic. Although the coronavirus pandemic has unleashed suffering across all countries, people in the developing world inevitably face greater challenges. They must contend with governments that are unable to provide support for the many people torn from sources of income; health systems that severely lack adequate personnel and equipment; massive capital flight; housing structures, especially in slums, that make lockdowns, quarantines, and social distancing impossible; and scapegoating of ethnic or religious minorities. Above all, the stark choice that the pandemic has forced upon states and societies is most acute for the citizens of the developing world: that between abiding by a lockdown to protect people's health and the need to work to put food on one's table. Not only is the effect of a lockdown more challenging in overcrowded conditions, but just as much, the sudden loss of income can be catastrophic for workers in developing countries who lack adequate welfare support. Furthermore, the political consequences of COVID-19 are arguably more severe for citizens of the developing world. Where illiberal populism reigns, not only is policy likely to be more erratic, it is also more likely that the pandemic serves as a cover for attacks on civil liberties.

In this chapter, we focus on the way the pandemic has deepened global inequalities by highlighting the unique struggles developing countries must deal with, as well as the ways in which particular communities and countries were made more vulnerable during the pandemic. We assess the macroeconomic picture in the developing world, as well as its relationship to the environment. We then analyze how the pandemic impacted different marginalized social groups — women, Indigenous Peoples, and ethnic, religious, and sexual minorities. Finally, we examine the illiberal and populist politics of three important developing countries that have had catastrophic results in handling the pandemic: India, Brazil, and the Philippines. These three countries arguably reflect the worst aspects of the pandemic: illiberal populist leadership that has led to spiralling deaths and infections. Brazil and India have the second- and third-largest number of deaths. Although the number of deaths is not as high as Brazil and India, the Philippines has the second-largest number of deaths in Southeast Asia despite having instituted one of the longest-lasting lockdowns in the world.

A Bleak Macroeconomic Picture in the Global South, but a Boost for the Environment?

COVID-19 resulted in the worst recession since the Second World War. The impact on the most vulnerable was severe: the crisis drove 70 to 100 million people into extreme poverty, to levels existing prior to 2017 (World Bank 2020). Interlinkages between domestic and international markets compounded economic effects in developing countries. Value chains were interrupted globally, negatively affecting key sectors in developing economies such as textiles, electronics, garments, and the automotive industry. Even exports of primary industrial commodities such as oil and metals were impacted.

In terms of sources of foreign capital, tourism decreased drastically, with tourist arrivals declining globally by up to 100 percent. Now, developing countries account for at least 30 percent of the world's tourism receipts. Capital outflows in developing countries during the first ninety days of the pandemic were 1.8 times higher (measured as a percentage of gross domestic product [GDP]) than such outflows during the first ninety days of the 2008 global financial crisis. In addition, foreign direct investment inflows dropped by 58 percent in 2020. The consequences of the above were disproportionately felt by the most vulnerable segments of the population, given the magnitude of informal employment in the value chain sectors and the large participation of women in the tourism workforce (75 percent of total workforce).

Moreover, the volume of remittances flowing to some developing regions decreased given the severe impact of the pandemic in advanced economies. Financial transfers from migrants working in advanced economies to their relatives in Sub-Saharan Africa decreased by 12.5 percent (including a 28 percent decline in Nigeria) and in East Asia and the Pacific by 7.9 percent. Significantly, remittances represent about 10 percent of the GDP of thirty low-to-middle-income-countries (LMICs). Considerably lower remittances have had drastic social consequences as these transfers help recipient families access health care, food, and other basic needs.

While the economic environment continued to be severely impacted into 2021, some recovery did occur and was expected to continue into 2022. Foreign direct investment in developing countries was estimated to increase by 10 to 15 percent, and a further potential increase in the following year could bring foreign direct investment to or close to the 2019 level. Furthermore, the global economy was estimated to grow 5.6 percent in 2021, with the developing world's GDP estimated to grow 4.4 percent.

As the chapter on the global economy also discusses, the effects of the economic turmoil will be long-lasting, given that the debt of governments and of corporations in developing countries was already at a high level and significantly greater than when the global financial crisis hit over a decade ago. On average, between 2007 and 2019, the debt of governments in developing countries increased by 11 percentage points of GDP, to reach 55.5 percent, and the debt of corporations increased 12 percentage points of GDP, to reach 39.8 percent. The high level of debt services thus places enormous stress on governments that need to focus on addressing critical domestic problems, and local currency devaluations and increased interest rates have raised the cost of debt. In addition, small- and middle-sized enterprises (SMEs), are facing high risks of bankruptcy.

In March 2020, the World Bank and the International Monetary Fund (IMF) asked bilateral creditors to suspend debt payments from countries requesting forbearance and the G20 agreed to a "debt standstill" from all official bilateral lenders for the 73 poorest and most vulnerable countries until at least the end of 2020. The suspension period was later agreed to be extended until December 2021. As of September 2021, only 40 eligible countries have participated in the initiative, with debt service relief totalling just US$5 billion. Furthermore, this temporary hiatus has little impact since private creditors are not as understanding. This is especially worrisome given the rise of private debt by non-financial corporations, which amounts to nearly three quarters of all debt in LMICs. Additionally, bilateral development aid, most of which was rerouted to COVID-related relief, has become harder to access.

As most governmental relief measures target formal workers and businesses (e.g., income replacement, supported furlough schemes, and tax relief) the socio-economic inequalities between the formal and the informal sector have the potential to become deeper in the long term. According to research conducted by the global network, Women in Informal Employment: Globalizing and Organizing (WIEGO 2020), the incomes of domestic workers, home-based workers, street vendors, and waste pickers were affected by the pandemic in five main ways: closing of public space, decrease in demand, rising costs of inputs, inability to access markets, and increase in childcare and eldercare responsibilities. With limited access to protective gear, medical insurance, and savings, many informal workers faced a stark dilemma in the crisis: die from hunger or die from the virus. In addition, rising unemployment in formal sectors drove many people into informal sectors of the economy, thereby increasing competition between already precarious businesses and workers. In countries where cash transfers are not universal and public policy responses are not gender-sensitive, the impacts will be long-lasting—especially given that when care work is included, around 80 percent of women in low-income countries work in the informal sector.

Despite the bleak economic picture painted above, the spread of COVID-19 has also brought reduced pressures on the natural environment across the globe. These "nature-positive" impacts give heart to those arguing that the current pandemic represents a once-in-a-lifetime opportunity to shift the global development paradigm towards a greener, more inclusive economy. As a result of the coronavirus outbreak's impact on travel and industry, many regions have experienced measurable drops in air pollution. Indeed, the impact of the coronavirus pandemic has been described by Paul Monk of the University of Leicester as the "largest scale experiment ever" into global air quality (Watts and Kommenda 2020). In terms of the world's deadliest air pollutant, fine particulate matter ($PM_{2.5}$) ten major global cities under lockdown (e.g., Delhi, London, Los Angeles, Milan, Mumbai, New York City, Rome, São Paulo, Seoul, and Wuhan) saw a drastic drop, by as much as 60 percent, in $PM_{2.5}$ pollution. As well, levels of nitrogen dioxide (NO_2) over cities and industrial clusters in Asia remained lower through 2020. Other air pollutants are on a similar track. Daily global carbon (CO_2) emissions in early April 2020 fell by 17 percent and could lead to an annual decline of up to 7 percent.

Water pollution has also been reduced in the beach areas of Bangladesh, Malaysia, Thailand, the Maldives, and Indonesia, with lockdowns and drops in tourism playing an important role. In October 2020 scientists reported, based on near-real-time activity data, an "unprecedented" abrupt 8.8 percent decrease in global CO_2 emissions in the first half of 2020 compared to the same period in 2019. More recently, in January 2021, it was reported that reductions in climate-related air pollution due to COVID-19 lockdowns in 2020 were larger than previously estimated. Of course, such declines are subject to post-pandemic rebounding, absent government intervention. The pandemic's greatest positive contribution to the struggle with climate change might be to prove that real drops in greenhouse gas (GHG) emissions are possible to achieve. COVID-19 may spur more concrete action than all the decades combined of global climate change talks.

A sharp increase in economic vulnerability will, in turn, increase pressure on forests to play a safety-net role: as more people among the rural poor turn to the forest for their subsistence needs and multinational companies for quick profits. In the Brazilian Amazon, deforestation increased by over 50 percent in early 2020. Further, a sustained drop in tourism revenues may alter the symbiotic relationship, which currently sustains people living close to wildlife and nature reserves where wealthier tourists abound.

Much of the global response to COVID-19 to date has been to view it as a medical challenge or an economic shock. Yet, COVID-19 and all preceding pandemics have their origins in nature, specifically in wildlife. Furthermore, all pandemics are linked to the changes that humans have made to the environment, especially as part of economic activity. For example, when we cut down a forest and replace it with a pig farm, the pigs risk exposure to a new virus and the threat to humans of another potential pandemic emerges. Intensive farming and lack of animal habitat are principally to blame. This is particularly the case in the South, where much of the world's biodiversity exists. But it is a crisis for the entire globe, as the driver of such unsustainable practices is the rise in demand for resources from both the North and the South.

The Pandemic's Impact on Marginalized Communities

The Effect on Women

The pandemic disproportionately affected marginalized groups in developing countries: women, Indigenous Peoples, and ethnic, religious, and sexual minorities. As in most previous crises, women and girls stand to suffer disproportionately from the health and economic shocks that COVID-19 presents. These challenges are global but are expected to be especially acute in LMICs where social services are lacking, informality reigns, and pre-existing gender gaps are wide. We stand to lose decades of progress in promoting gender equality and women's empowerment.

One of the earliest impacts of the pandemic was the shock to labour markets induced by reduced consumer demand, supply chain considerations, and non-pharmaceutical interventions such as lockdowns, work from home directives, and social distancing practices in the workplace. Here, there were several factors at play affecting women's experience in a COVID-19 labour market. The International Labour Organization (ILO) confirms that women tend to be disproportionately represented in public-facing and high-risk occupations such as food services, tourism and hospitality services, education, and frontline care work. This means that their jobs are either more likely to be cut by lockdown or are considered essential. Those who have maintained employment have done so out of necessity in the informal sector with poor sanitary conditions and for those in essential public-facing occupations, such as food services and health care, at heightened risk of contracting the illness. Reports from the World Health Organization (WHO) and other organizations have already noted increased stigma and violence against community health workers who are seen as vectors of disease, adding mental health and stress to workplace hazards.

With lockdowns and economic contraction, school and daycare closures, women are already shouldering a disproportionate amount of unpaid care responsibilities. One reason has to do with women's lower average earnings than men, so that in families without lockdown induced job losses, it is less costly for the women to withdraw from the workforce to care for their children. The health crisis has also led to an increased need for care of the sick and older population, which likely also falls on the shoulder of women. If the economy is to restart, finding safe and reliable care options will be a necessary condition, and there is a concern that the care economy, largely offered by the private or non-governmental organization (NGO) sectors in the Global South, is on the verge of collapse. Many households will have little choice but to entrust the care of the young to older siblings, with potentially devastating implications for girls' schooling and thus long-term well-being. Any reopening strategy will need to consider childcare and schooling as an essential service (WEDLab 2020).

A major concern brought about by increased isolation during COVID-19 lockdowns, financial hardship, and increased stress, was the acute increase in violence against women and children (VAWC). There is already a considerably large body of evidence of a sharp increase in VAWC globally, including concerns of increases in child marriages. And this volume of evidence was gathered despite increased difficulties in collecting data, as face-to-face surveys have stopped and phone interviews make it difficult to ensure respondents' confidentiality (Peterman, Bhatia, and Guedes 2020), and women's prolonged isolation with their abusers mean they are less likely to report abuse.

The Effect on Indigenous Peoples

In spite of their many differences, Indigenous Peoples across the globe are disadvantaged on a number of social and economic indicators compared to their non-Indigenous counterparts. As Danielle DeLuca

(2020) of the NGO Cultural Survival succinctly put it, "We know that coronavirus does not discriminate, but we know that societies do." Indigenous Peoples have suffered centuries of discrimination and COVID-19 presents a new threat to their health and survival, given they are already more prone to infectious disease. Prospects for such communities in many parts of the world will remain at best challenging as Indigenous Peoples continue to struggle with food and water insecurity, lack of access to health care, encroachment on traditional lands, and continuing human rights violations.

Within Indigenous communities, Elders are particularly vulnerable, given age is one of the main factors associated with the severity of the disease. This has significant implications for Indigenous communities, since Elders play a key role as holders of traditional knowledge and practices—including conservation of biodiversity, upholding traditions and customs, and serving as custodians of customary law and governance.

The extent of the current and future impact on Indigenous Peoples is uncertain as in most other population groups. However, some preliminary figures are troubling. In Brazil, for example, the organization Articulation of Indigenous Peoples of Brazil reports that 9.1 percent of Indigenous People who contract the disease are dying, nearly double the 5.2 percent rate among the general Brazilian population (APIB 2020). Absent reliable and consistent information across the globe on the pandemic-Indigenous relationship means it will be doubly difficult for countries and Indigenous groups to mitigate the health and socioeconomic effects of COVID-19.

Food insecurity among Indigenous communities is growing as prices of basic food items rise and the scarcity and price of seeds for planting increases in some regions. National governments' enforced countrywide lockdowns (ranging from Guatemala, to India, to Nepal) mean Indigenous farmers have been unable to tend to their crops.

Since first contact, Indigenous communities have had to cope with infection and disease transmitted from sources outside their own regions. In the case of COVID-19, as in past events, Indigenous communities are proving resilient and resourceful. Indeed, traditional Indigenous practices such as sealing off communities and voluntary isolation have been adopted with promising results by non-Indigenous societies across the globe—in both rural and urban settings and in countries of the South and North. Traditional knowledge and methods of healing could improve Indigenous Peoples' resiliency.

Indigenous communities and organizations are already helping one another, as understanding of the virus and its spread in traditional lands and territories improves and Indigenous-appropriate mitigation and treatment methods are developed.

The Effect on Ethnic, Religious, and Sexual Minorities

COVID-19 has also had a broad range of disproportionate and adverse impacts upon ethnic, racial, religious, and sexual minority communities. Death rates for some of these communities have reportedly been several times higher than other groups. For example, at the beginning of the crisis, it was already found that in Brazil's São Paulo State, people of colour are 62 percent more likely to die from COVID-19 than their white counterparts (Genot 2020). Countermeasures such as lockdowns are having particularly severe effects on racialized groups. While reliable data are unavailable in most countries, the Brookings Institution determined that in the first three months of the crisis in the United States, 1,013 white people died, compared to 1,448 Black people, and 1,698 Hispanic/Latino people (Ford et al. 2020).

In many regions of the North and South, ethnic minorities work in at-risk and low-paid jobs, which leave them more exposed to COVID-19 and other diseases. Now there is growing recognition that these same people are serving in essential services on the frontline in the fight against COVID-19. Filipino nurses in the United States have been particularly hard hit by the pandemic. One survey by a nurses' union, National Nurses United, estimates that one third of nurses who have died due to COVID-19 are Filipinos (Powell 2021). In Guyana, the Ministry of Health has created awareness videos to support the frontline workforce in non-medical activities in minority and Indigenous languages.

Lesbian, gay, bisexual, transgender, and intersex (LGBTI) individuals are proving more vulnerable than most. People living with compromised immune systems (e.g., HIV/AIDS) face greater risks from COVID-19, as do people experiencing homelessness (many of whom are LGTBI people) who are less able to protect themselves through physical distancing and safe hygiene practices. Healthcare discrimination further increases their risk from COVID-19. LGBTI people are often the least protected minority communities under law, and it is no surprise that homophobic and transphobic rhetoric is amplifying in countries such as Uganda, the Cayman Islands, Panama, and Iraq.

Scapegoating of religious minorities is also on the rise during the pandemic—paralleling (similarly baseless) accusations against religious minorities during the Great Plague of Europe (1347–1351). During COVID-19, religious minorities in a wide range of countries are being blamed for the spread of the disease. Hindus in Pakistan, Muslims in India, Yazidis and Kakais in Iraq, Shia in Saudi Arabia, and Jews in France and Iran have all been targeted.

Populism, Inequality, and the Coronavirus

In countries where illiberal populist leaders govern, the response to COVID-19 has been especially weak—driven by a failure to follow public health guidelines, erratic policy, machismo rhetoric, and scapegoating of a host of groups. But when illiberal populism combines with deep-seated poverty, as it does in the developing world, the results are truly devastating. In India, Brazil, and the Philippines, where COVID-19 struck during the tenure of illiberal leaders, the results have included catastrophic health outcomes, economic collapse, and deepening repression—in effect, a perfect storm for a complete decline in development writ large, or, in Amartya Sen's words, of "development as freedom."

India

India has been one of the countries hardest hit by the pandemic. As of December 2021, it had the third-highest number of deaths and the second-highest number of infections (in fact, the highest number of infections in the developing world). Its response to the pandemic was characterized by one of the most stringent lockdowns, scapegoating of the country's Muslim minority, and minimal public support for the most precarious groups—particularly workers in the informal economy. India's first lockdown was imposed within four hours of its announcement and lasted seven weeks. While a lockdown is challenging for all citizens, its impact on the working class and poor was especially acute. Not only do the urban poor live cheek to jowl in ramshackle abodes, thereby making social distancing close to impossible, they also earn their income through daily wages that are crucial in order to put food on the table and to cover rent. Under lockdown, individuals without much savings were physically and financially trapped. As a result of the lockdown, millions of urban migrants decided to head back to their villages leading to desperate scenes of individuals walking down highways in scorching heat and stories of migrants being killed on the highway. What India's prime minister Narendra Modi did not foresee was the sense in which urban informal workers would feel completely trapped under lockdown and seek to exit. Here, the most vulnerable could not escape large crowds nor could they maintain their livelihoods. Analysts now point to this lockdown—seen as "too tight and too porous" as the cause of India's economic decline and extensive spread of the coronavirus (Gettleman 2020). In 2020, the Indian economy declined by 7.3 percent, with 200 million people expected to fall into poverty.

India suffered even more when the second wave of COVID-19 struck the country in April 2021. For several months in spring, India grabbed global headlines as a country ripping at the seams, accounting for more than half the infections in the world and some 400,000 cases per day. By the end of May, more than 300,000 people had lost their lives. Independent studies projected that the real death toll was at least twice as high as what the government reported (Gamio and Glanz 2021). This second wave occurred in large part because the Modi government proclaimed victory too early, with the health minister asserting that they were at the "endgame" of the pandemic, and political and religious mass gatherings were allowed again. The result was a country overwhelmed for several months by a second wave that devastated every corner of India.

Along with government failure to prevent the second wave's devastation, the pandemic had also provided the government an opportunity to scapegoat religious minorities. An Islamic missionary movement, Tablighi Jamaat, held a large congregation in a slum area in early March 2020 that acted as a super-spreader event. Indian health officials estimated that one third of the country's cases were linked to the group's congregation. As a result, Muslims have been assaulted and beaten in cities and villages. Right-wing Hindu groups labelled the Tablighi Jamaat "criminal" with a politician from the Bharatiya Janata Party calling it "corona terrorism." Right-wing Hindu groups distributed saffron-coloured flags to distinguish Hindu market vendors following rumours that Muslims were purposely contaminating food with the virus. On social media, hashtags such as #CoronaJihad and #TablighiVirus began trending throughout the country. #CoronaJihad was the top trending hashtag on Twitter for several days. Fake news circulated that Muslims were spreading the virus by spitting on fruits, licking utensils, sneezing in unison, and spitting at police officers to escape quarantine. Sikh temples in the state of Punjab sent out messages warning people not to purchase milk from Muslims because it was infected with coronavirus. "One of the key features of anti-Muslim sentiment in India for quite a long time has been the idea that Muslims themselves are a kind of infection in the body politic," noted Arjun Appadurai. "So there's a kind of affinity between this long-standing image and the new anxieties surrounding coronavirus" (Perrigo 2020).

The Modi government has furthermore used the crisis to continue its crackdown on Muslims, following the passage of the discriminatory Citizenship Amendment Act in December 2019, which established religion as a basis for granting citizenship. In the early months of the outbreak of COVID-19, the government questioned, detained, and arrested at least 50 Muslim activists and lawyers.

Brazil

After the United States, Brazil has the highest number of deaths during the pandemic. Among all countries in the developing world, Brazil's response to the coronavirus crisis stands out as arguably the worst. President Jair Bolsonaro initially dismissed COVID-19 as a "little flu." He openly flouted public health regulations, attended many rallies without a mask until a judge ordered him to wear one, and issued a decree that allowed hairdressers and gyms to be considered essential businesses and therefore be allowed to reopen. In open conflict with his health ministers, Bolsonaro ousted two of them at the height of the pandemic. Bolsonaro also pushed the health ministry to issue guidelines that recommend the use of antimalarial drug hydroxychloroquine and ordered military labs to increase production.

Challenged from across the political spectrum for a lacklustre response to the pandemic, Bolsonaro waged an attack on Brazil's institutions—Congress, the courts, the media, mayors, and governors. As the number of infected and deaths rose sharply by June 2020, putting Brazil on track as second only to the United States in number of deaths, the Brazilian government decided it would no longer publish the full extent of data, limiting its reporting to the number of new daily cases and fatalities. Bolsonaro claimed that the data being produced until then were flawed anyway. This was a blatant attempt to obfuscate the severity of the pandemic, precisely when Brazil's tallies were rising so sharply.

In response to Bolsonaro's callous attitude toward the pandemic, Brazilian citizens and opposition politicians pushed back. Governors and mayors refused to follow Bolsonaro's directive to open hair salons and gyms and put forth their own strict regulations of social distancing. In major cities throughout the country, *panelaços*—banging pots and pans as a form of protest—broke out, with cries of *Fora Bolsonaro* ("get out Bolsonaro") as a way of expressing intense discontent with the president's handling of the coronavirus crisis. Even some of the wealthier neighbourhoods of Rio de Janeiro, where Bolsonaro had significant support in the 2018 election, joined the *panelaços*.

In October 2021, the Brazilian Senate approved a 1,200-page report that charged Bolsonaro and other government officials with crimes against humanity and for "deliberately" exposing the country to the risk of a pandemic. The report emphasizes egregious government conduct, including "the delay in purchasing vaccines, false statements about the virus, the campaign for unproven medical treatments, and the belief that obtaining herd immunity through widespread infection was the best solution" (Alves 2021). Scathing in its criticism, the report documents the government's callousness and unprofessionalism: while Pfizer sent over 100 emails on the availability of its vaccine, the government never replied. Furthermore, the charge of crimes against humanity is explicitly linked to Bolsonaro's anti-Indigenous policies. With Indigenous Peoples already under attack since the beginning of Bolsonaro's administration, the pandemic wrought even greater devastation on Indigenous communities. The report thus sought to bring justice to a country where the mortality rate was five times higher than the global average.

The Philippines

President Rodrigo Duterte engaged the COVID-19 pandemic with the same iron-fisted machismo as that of his signature policy, the ruthless war on drugs. After the Philippine Department of Health reported the first case of COVID-19 in the country on 30 January 2020 from a Chinese national, and later on 7 March, the first local transmission of COVID-19, Duterte put in place one of the "fiercest and longest-lasting" lockdowns (*The Economist* 2020). Named "Enhanced Community Quarantine" (ECQ), the scheme covered the entire island of Luzon—the biggest island of the archipelago and its capital Manila—as well as other smaller islands, accounting altogether for about half of its 105 million people. Implementation was drastic and arbitrary: 100,000 individuals were fined and even arrested for minor infractions, such as forgetting to use a mask. Faithful to his political style, Duterte went as far as declaring that the armed forces and police should shoot dead those violating confinement policies. As measured by the Oxford Blavatnik School's "stringency index"—a composite measure on strictness of lockdown policies, including school closures, workplace closures, and travel bans—the Philippines had one of the highest indices throughout the pandemic, especially in April and May 2020. Its lockdowns have continued, almost non-stop, in a bewildering variety of forms, termed as "enhanced quarantine."

Yet despite one of the harshest lockdowns, the Philippines had the second-highest number of people infected in Southeast Asia. This reflects the country's failure to address other crucial policy responses to the pandemic, such as effective testing, tracing, and vaccine delivery. Furthermore, with millions losing their jobs, by August 2020, the country had entered into a recession—the first in three decades—registering a quarterly decline in GDP of 16.5 percent. Although the economy was expected to grow by 4 or 5 percentage points in 2021, in 2020 it registered a 9.6 percent decline. Economic Planning Secretary, Karl Kendrick Chua, estimated that it would take ten years before the country returned to pre-pandemic growth levels.

Notwithstanding discontent regarding what is in effect an *ad hoc* and improvised response, Duterte continued to enjoy the support of many members of Congress and of the middle class, including the large Philippine diaspora. With his control assured in the House of Representatives, the Senate, and the Supreme Court, and in the context of COVID-19, Duterte pushed the adoption of a new anti-terrorist law, which includes a number of measures that under the guise of fighting back terrorism can curtail democratic and political rights. Philippines human rights advocates even compared the recent Anti-Terrorist Act to Hong Kong's new national security law.

Whether Duterte will maintain his stratospherically high popularity ratings, however, is still not clear. The sharp decline of the Philippine economy puts the country in one of its worst states in decades. As Solita Monsod, a prominent Philippine economist and former head of the National and Economic Development Authority observed: "Never before, not even in the country's debt crisis under [president] Ferdinand Marcos, has [the economy] performed so poorly" (Castaneda 2020).

The Future of the Developing World in the Age of COVID-19

We close by emphasizing three key points regarding the future of the developing world in an age marked by COVID-19. First, we note the *urgency of increasing financial support for the developing world*, but also the difficulties therein. Canada has played an important role in seeking remedies in the developing world as the co-chair of the "Initiative for Financing for Development in the Era of COVID-19 and Beyond," where at a meeting in September 2020, it pledged $400 million in development and humanitarian aid to fight the pandemic. Overall, however, the actual global deliverables of development aid have been of limited scope. Weak economic situations have not allowed most developing countries to launch sizeable emergency packages, which averaged only 5.4 percent of GDP. Multilateral development banks announced large financing volumes. However, a relevant proportion of their support to the public sector is still yet to be disbursed, and the approach to support the private sector has mostly been focused on financing banks, which has an uncertain effect. In addition, the G20's agreement to suspend debt payments from the poorest and most vulnerable countries will be insufficient unless such an initiative is extended over the next years, accompanied by debt restructurings, and joined by private creditors and multilateral development banks.

In the broader and longer term, it is difficult to forecast the impact of COVID-19 on development policy and international cooperation. The pandemic exposed and, indeed, deepened existing inequalities both within and among countries. The discovery of a new coronavirus variant, Omicron, in southern Africa in November 2021 highlighted the deep disadvantages that poor nations face. Despite the initiatives of UN-led COVAX to provide more equitable access to vaccines, Africa had only 10 percent of its population vaccinated with one dose when the Omicron variant burst on the scene. The response of Western nations was one of closing borders rather than expressing solidarity with African nations or seeking a more expedited and just distribution of vaccines.

Two trends can thus be delineated within the context of what, at least in part, can be characterized as a crisis in globalization. One track is for countries to pull further away from regional and global connectedness. The immediate response to Omicron would appear to reflect that. The other is to seize the moment and build back a stronger, fairer globalized system supporting international development cooperation. Fundamental shifts in policy have yet to be introduced by countries and institutions, given that both the developed and developing worlds remain in crisis mode. However, it is not implausible that COVID-19 will compel radical shifts in policy and delivery—as major crises in the past have engendered.

Our second concluding observation is that a general pattern has emerged in both *developing and industrialized* economies: it is the most marginalized communities—Indigenous Peoples in the Brazilian Amazon, the African American and Latino communities, as well as Filipino nurses in the United States, religious minorities in India, immigrant groups in France—that are being most devastated by the pandemic. The pandemic has thus torn through the weakest social fabric across the globe, demonstrating clearly how health status, social structure, and economic livelihoods are so intertwined. It is these *marginalized social groups and communities that must be given priority* as we search for effective policy solutions.

Finally, we argue that although much of what has been discussed here is quite pessimistic, we also should see this pandemic as an opportunity for moving beyond the "old normal"—an old normal that takes for granted people's callous relationship with nature, including especially wildlife; that dismisses the conditions of the developing world as largely irrelevant to the health and welfare of lives in the rich and industrialized nations; and that puts minimal faith in the potential and need for global cooperation. While we have rejected the idea that this pandemic's virus is blind to social and political context—that it is an "equalizer"—we end by observing that the deep linkages between developed and developing countries make it absolutely imperative that *the countries of the North invest intellectually, financially, and humanely in improving the inequitable conditions that plague the South* and its ties to the North. In an ironic twist, the North could be compelled to invest in prevention of root causes of developmental dilemmas in the South as high-income countries suffer great monetary losses. A response to new coronavirus variants, such as Omicron, that are rooted in solidarity will in the long-run yield better economic and public health outcomes for the richer nations. Ultimately, the response to the pandemic must take on a larger ethical vision that sees universal ties as crucial to effective policy.

References

Alves, Lisa. 2021. "Health Experts Welcome Brazil COVID-19 Inquiry Findings." *The Lancet* 398, no. 10312 (November 6): 1674–1675.

APIB (Articulation of Indigenous Peoples of Brazil). 2020. "Indigenous Lives and Covid-19" Newsletter 1, May 14. https://apiboficial.org/2020/05/14/01-indigenous-lives-and-covid-19/?lang=en.

Castaneda, Jason. 2020. "Duterte Tightens Grip, as the Philippines Falls Apart." *AsiaTimes*, September 24, 2020. https://asiatimes.com/2020/09/duterte-tightens-grip-as-the-philippines-falls-apart/.

DeLuca, Danielle. "COVID-19's Growing Impact on Indigenous Communities Globally." Cultural Survival. April 9, 2020. https://www.culturalsurvival.org/news/covid-19s-growing-impact-indigenous-communities-globally.

The Economist. 2020. "The Philippines' Fierce Lockdown Drags On, despite Uncertain Benefits." July 11, 2020. https://www.economist.com/asia/2020/07/11/the-philippines-fierce-lockdown-drags-on-despite-uncertain-benefits.

Ford, Tiffany N., Sarah Reber, and Richard R. Reeves. 2020. "Race Gaps in COVID-19 Deaths Are Even Bigger than They Appear." *Brookings Institution*, June 16, 2020. https://www.brookings.edu/blog/up-front/2020/06/16/race-gaps-in-covid-19-deaths-are-even-bigger-than-they-appear/.

Friedman, Thomas L. 2005. *The World Is Flat.* New York: Farrar, Straus and Giroux.

Gamio, Lazaro, and James Glanz. 2021. "Just How Big Could India's True Covid Toll Be?" *The New York Times*, May 25, 2021. https://www.nytimes.com/interactive/2021/05/25/world/asia/india-covid-death-estimates.html.

Genot, Louis. 2020. "In Brazil, Coronavirus Hits Blacks Harder than Whites." *Agence France Presse*, May 7, 2020. https://www.barrons.com/news/in-brazil-coronavirus-hits-blacks-harder-than-whites-01588886404.

Gettleman, Jeffrey. 2020. "Coronavirus Crisis Shatters India's Big Dreams." *The New York Times*, September 5, 2020. https://www.nytimes.com/2020/09/05/world/asia/india-economy-coronavirus.html.

Perrigo, Billy. 2020. "It Was Already Dangerous to Be Muslim in India. Then Came the Coronavirus." *Time*, April 3, 2020. https://time.com/5815264/coronavirus-india-islamophobia-coronajihad/.

Peterman, Amber, Amiya Bhatia, and Alessandra Guedes. 2020. "Remote Data Collection on Violence against Women during COVID-19." UNICEF, May 29, 2020. https://www.unicef-irc.org/article/1997-remote-data-collection-on-violence-against-women-during-covid-19-a-conversation-with.html.

Powell, Luca. 2021. "'It's Starting Again': Why Filipino Nurses Dread the Second Wave." *The New York Times*, January 15, 2021. https://www.nytimes.com/2021/01/15/nyregion/filipino-nurses-coronavirus.html.

Watts, Jonathan, and Niko Kommenda. 2020. "Coronavirus Pandemic Leading to Huge Drop in Air Pollution." *The Guardian*, March 23, 2020. https://www.theguardian.com/environment/2020/mar/23/coronavirus-pandemic-leading-to-huge-drop-in-air-pollution.

WEDLab, Institute for the Study of International Development, McGill University. 2020. "COVID-19 and the Care Economy in the Global South." Webinar Summary. June 11. http://womensempowerment.lab.mcgill.ca/seminars/care-economy-global-south/.

WIEGO (Women in Informal Employment: Globalizing and Organizing). 2020. *Informal Workers in the COVID-19 Crisis: A Global Picture of Sudden Impact and Long-Term Risk*. Manchester: WIEGO. https://www.wiego.org/sites/default/files/resources/file/Informal%20Workers%20in%20the%20COVID-19%20Crisis_WIEGO_July_2020.pdf.

World Bank. 2020. *Global Economic Prospects*. Washington, D.C.: World Bank.

CHAPTER 10

Migration and Citizenship

Magdalena Dembińska, Valérie Amiraux, François Crépeau,
Alain Gagnon, Mireille Paquet, Thomas Soehl, and Luna Vives

In mid-2020, the United Nations (UN) estimated that there were 281 million international migrants across all categories. While almost two thirds of these people settled in another country for work, this population is highly heterogeneous and includes students, asylum seekers, families and isolated individuals (both adults and minors), seasonal agricultural workers, and highly skilled employees, as well as non-status persons.

During the pandemic, limiting human mobility emerged as a global mitigation measure, first when international borders were closed (entry bans, airport closures), then when various entry restrictions or conditions were implemented in most countries. In March 2021, these were estimated at nearly 108,000 worldwide (IOM 2021). In addition to border controls, the pandemic accentuated migrants' multidimensional precarity within their countries of residence, notably through the tightening of political and legal instruments governing their stay.

This chapter looks at the relationship between Canada and the rest of the world, examining the repressive role of borders during the pandemic and the precarity of migrants, focusing on the situation of three groups: migrant healthcare workers, seasonal agricultural workers, and international students. Although migrants were in a precarious situation even before the pandemic, the pandemic exacerbated its brutality and amplified its effects.

Migrant Control and Precarity: The Role of Borders

The role of borders in controlling migrants is a field of study in its own right (Wilson and Donnan 2012). The notion of a border regime underlines the changing nature of borders: "migrants face multiple border interfaces that aim to 'filter' them—beyond the linear border (remote control), within it (national controls) and on its very route (official crossing points)" (Bassi and Souiah 2019, 10). The COVID-19-induced crisis has led to an updated regime. In April 2020, the lockdowns (i.e., internal mobility controls) and the decision by a majority of states to—indefinitely—suspend non-essential international arrivals to their countries (91 percent of the world's population resided in these countries at that time) or to close their borders entirely to non-citizens and non-residents (39 percent of the world's population resided in these countries at that time) took border "securitization" measures—albeit, with unprecedented impermeability—with which experts are very familiar (Pew Research Centre 2020). There is no doubt that the pandemic restructured the hierarchy of ways migrant mobility is controlled—in the name of contagion—taking restrictive measures that prioritize national borders. The militarization of borders continued, in the Mediterranean and in the United States, Pakistan, and India; and legal instruments for protecting vulnerable people, particularly the principle of *non-refoulement*, were suspended. Some countries closed their doors to migrant ships in distress and rescue boats, failing their marine safety duties. Meanwhile, in Asia and Latin America, thousands of migrants were forced (by government orders or a lack of employment) to return to their home countries, in a kind of "great return," which further spread the pandemic to countries that were little affected but have fragile health systems (e.g., Guatemala and Venezuela).

The infringement of fundamental rights associated with migration and refugee protection did not begin with the pandemic (see chapter 8). For example, the antagonism between national and international jurisdictions has grown over the past 15 years, with the former pledging to protect against the "risks" associated with immigration, notably by intensifying border controls and mobility restrictions; the latter arguing for respect for human rights irrespective of individuals' nationality, to consider cooperation-based international migration governance. The Global Compact on Migration adopted in December 2018 by the UN is a case in point. The number of migrants has increased significantly since 2000, and the public policies of states have become more resistant to individual mobility (with the exception of certain elites). The pandemic has only reinforced these tensions and exacerbated the precarity of the most vulnerable.

Precarity is a "politically induced condition in which certain populations experience a lack of social and economic support networks" that puts them at an increased risk of "disease, poverty, starvation, displacement and violence" (Butler 2009, 25–26). It encompasses both a lack of protection and socioeconomic instability, and it affects individuals and groups differently according to interrelated factors, such as gender, race, class, age, or migration status. If mobility is a universal right, the immobility imposed by lockdown policies is a striking revelation of the singular vulnerability of migrants.

Several situations come to mind to illustrate the unequal precarity in respecting health measures. Migrant-intake centres and refugee camps (e.g., the Moria camp in Greece that was ravaged by fire in September 2020) are places where living conditions—unacceptable outside the context of the pandemic—make following health measures illogical, if not ridiculous. The concentration of migrants in some so-called essential sectors (e.g., health and agriculture) exposed them disproportionately to disease in both Canada and Northern Europe, where one in five workers is a migrant worker (ILO 2017). The many outbreaks in slaughterhouses or workers' hostels highlight this. Official health department figures document the cases in Saudi Arabia and Singapore: in the former, 75 percent of new cases confirmed as of May 7, 2020, were migrants; in the latter, over 95 percent of cases confirmed as of June 19, 2020, were migrants, and over 93 percent of these cases were the result of overcrowding in accommodation dormitories (Migration Data Portal 2023).

Part of sovereign states' central function is to limit the precarity of those residing in their countries and particularly citizens. The allocation of privileges and precarious regimes is based largely on borders, sovereignty, and citizenship status. For example, in terms of international protection regimes, precarity does not justify refugee status or access to rights in a foreign country. Historically, rich countries that attract immigrants—whether in the North or South—depend on the comparative advantage provided in large part by migrant workers, of which the slave, the bonded labourer, and the seasonal worker are just a few examples.

In 2020, the insecurity experienced by these workers, who are frequently employed in sectors perceived as "dirty, dangerous and humiliating" with particularly grueling working conditions, is often linked to the fact that they are not only at the mercy of their employers but that they are also excluded from rights-protection systems. What makes this precarity even more ironic is that migrant workers' jobs help grow their host countries' economies and empower their citizens. Many studies have shown how heavily several economic sectors rely on the constant presence of migrant workers (e.g., agriculture, construction, hospitality, healthcare, and childcare). During the pandemic, these sectors emerged from obscurity and became "essential," with no changes to workers' precarious conditions.

Legal insecurity compounds this economic insecurity, often because of the temporary nature of migrants' administrative status. Temporary immigration status generally does not give these individuals access to the rights and social protections available to residents. As a result, the living conditions of these migrants depend largely on the discretionary—and sometimes arbitrary—decisions of states and key players, such as recruiters, employers, educational institutions, and employment agencies.

Over the past 25 years, temporary statuses—initially developed for specific economic sectors—have been used more and more in a wide range of cases, from international students to asylum seekers. In so-called "immigration countries," national permanent immigration systems have often become two-step programs (Dauvergne 2016). To qualify for permanent status, a person first needs a temporary permit. In countries that offer little or no permanent status (e.g., Gulf countries), the temporary condition can sometimes last a lifetime (Boucher and Gest 2018).

The growing prominence of these temporary statuses has given rise to a sort of "second-class citizen," whose life is precarious in a number of ways, often associating social class, gender, and race with migratory status. For example, in the countries of the Global South, "expatriates" from the Global North are often treated far better than "migrant workers," despite frequently holding the same residence permits, as they benefit from superior social capital. For these migrants, the pre-pandemic world was already largely riddled with precarity, with borders playing a central role in the distribution of privileges and access to rights and social protection. To better understand the pandemic's impacts on migrants in a country like Canada, it is essential to look back at their administrative situations and describe the bureau-cratic conditions of their legal—and therefore social—vulnerabilities.

Migrant Workers: Health and Agriculture

So-called "essential" jobs—with their dangerous and arduous work-ing conditions and low pay—are disproportionately held by tem-porary workers or asylum seekers, despite a permanent or recurring need for labour in these sectors. In Canada, workers primarily obtain work permits under the Temporary Foreign Worker Program (TFWP) or the International Mobility Program—two programs designed to address short-term labour shortages.

These workers rarely benefit from equal treatment in the work-place and often have trouble accessing social rights. Their work per-mits are generally "closed" (i.e., associated with a single employer). Often, if they lose their job, they lose their status and permission to reside in Canada. Therefore, the employer holds extraordinary power, which explains why migrant workers fear losing their jobs if they speak up or report abuse. Most of the time, workers are recruited by temporary employment agencies that charge recruitment fees, despite this practice being prohibited. Because workers are not recruited by the employer directly, workplace safety obligations are sometimes opaque.

Although migrant workers contribute to the Canada Pension Plan or Employment Insurance benefits, they do not have access to public subsidy programs (e.g., the Canadian Emergency Response Benefit [CERB] introduced during the pandemic) if they lose their status. This is not only the case for international workers but also for students whose social insurance number expired at the end of their visa. The closure of visa processing centres significantly slowed the residence permit renewal process. For those awaiting status, accepting unreported employment was sometimes the only option for making ends meet. Following demands from various migrant-support organi-zations, foreigners who lost their temporary resident status during the COVID-19 pandemic were granted additional time to regain it. This temporary measure does not remove the demand for stable immigra-tion status for all these workers, particularly in the agricultural and healthcare sectors.

In Quebec, 20 percent of those infected with COVID-19 were healthcare workers, including many legal immigrants and asylum seekers. Numerous cases of migrant families infected by the virus while working in the province's long-term care facilities (CHSLD) were reported in the media. These migrant workers were on the front lines in the fight against the spread of the virus, yet were among the most vulnerable.

With worldwide shortages of healthcare personnel, these workers are in demand in Canada and elsewhere. The demand for orderlies and other care staff increases as populations age because long-term care involves providing daily assistance to people, either in their own homes or in residences. The High-Level Commission on Health Employment and Economic Growth set up by the UN and the Organisation for Economic Co-operation and Development (OECD) estimates that—by 2030—there will be a shortfall of 18 million workers in the healthcare sector (OECD 2020). Migrants are overrepresented in the health and social services sectors in many countries. According to OECD data (2019), the healthcare services of the United States, the United Kingdom, France, Spain, Italy, Germany, and the Czech Republic depend on foreign-born workers, from orderlies and nurses to doctors (OECD 2020). Traditionally, rich countries' resistance to the migration of foreign-trained healthcare workers is the result of cor-poratism aimed at protecting the jobs and income levels of domestic healthcare workers, particularly doctors; a fear that these workers do not have the skill level required; and an ethical concern about depriving the countries of origin of their employees. However, to remedy the shortage of healthcare workers, the World Health Organization (WHO) recommends increasing their mobility (WHO 2010).

Immigration systems often favour highly educated workers, such as doctors and nurses. However, many healthcare workers, such as orderlies, are considered "low-skilled," thereby making them ineligible for permanent resident visas. The low pay of these jobs is also a problem. In February 2020—just weeks before the start of the pandemic—the United Kingdom unveiled a new points-based immigration policy to regulate post-Brexit migration. With some exceptions (if the government felt there was a labour shortage in a particular sector), the minimum annual income threshold to qualify for immigration was set at £25,000. Such a requirement applies to many healthcare workers now considered "essential," including paramedics, nurses, caregivers, and midwives. During the pandemic, visas for doctors, nurses, and paramedics that expired before 1 October 2020 were extended automatically for a year.

In agriculture, migrants take jobs that citizens and permanent residents shy away from because of their arduous nature and low pay. For example, in Quebec, a farm worker's salary is lower than the average wage—it is only beneficial if compared to the average wages in the country of origin or to the unemployment that would await migrant workers there. Agricultural work is known as "3D"—difficult, dirty, and dangerous. The hours are long, the days hot, and the harvest cannot be postponed. Often housed in barracks on the farm, migrant workers are socially isolated. They live and work on farms far from urban areas with virtually non-existent means of transport. This limits their ability to communicate with the outside world, and the fact that they live on private land accessible only with the owner's permission limits the ability of organizations (e.g., NGOs, associations, and trade unions) to help them. The argument that "migrant workers do work that citizens and permanent residents don't want to do," and that—therefore—it is essential to recruit a temporary workforce, is patently false. The need for agricultural labour is permanent, and greenhouse production means that farming is no longer seasonal. If wages and working conditions were negotiated properly, agricultural workers could be recruited among citizens and permanent residents, including those from an immigrant background. A "standardized" agricultural labour market would reduce the number of temporary migrant workers and increase the price of agricultural products, as was the case in industry when the labour force was unionized at the beginning of the twentieth century. This means that authorities would need to plan a medium- to long-term transition and implement compensatory measures to avoid a farming collapse, which would require real political will.

Farm workers' situation is the result of a combination of a migration policy that creates a highly precarious administrative status and a lack of investment in the oversight of the application of labour and occupational health and safety standards. To keep employment costs as low as possible, farmers most often employ either non-status migrant workers or migrant workers who are part of the Seasonal Agricultural Worker Program (SAWP) or the agricultural component of the TFWP. Because of these programs, some 25,000 people from Mexico and the West Indies travel to Canada each year to work on Canadian farms temporarily. The SAWP contains several guarantees for migrant workers, many of which the TFWP lacks.

However, these programs have major flaws, including the closed work permit and the role of agencies. In particular, in Quebec and Ontario, farm workers do not have the right to unionize and collectively bargain their working conditions. The Supreme Court of Canada endorsed this situation in the Fraser case,[1] when it affirmed that it was important for workers to be able to join associations and make representations to employers, but that this did not include a right to form unions and bargain collectively. This decision makes no mention of the fact that most of the workers concerned are migrants with precarious status.

The ban on unions severely limits the pressure workers can exert to improve their working conditions and encourages employers to retaliate against individuals who are considered "troublemakers." Those who complain or try to form associations are often fired, or their names are added to a "blacklist" that is sent to their consulate so that they cannot be rehired. Moreover, labour inspections on farms are rare. There is insufficient oversight by authorities of working conditions, workplace health and safety, housing, food, and access to healthcare: every year the media reports horror stories about migrant workers' conditions on certain farms.

From this perspective, the COVID-19 pandemic did not help. "Essential" farm workers were recruited and given visas, but their "essential" status had no impact on their precarious status or working conditions. Worse still, they were often forced to work without protective equipment or measures (e.g., masks, gloves, testing, preventive withdrawal). Canadians were protected by requiring migrant workers to be quarantined on arrival, but the measures required to protect migrants' health were not implemented.

Migrant workers' precarious situation is not unique to Canada or to northern countries. The same is true of South–South migrants and refugees (migration that has outnumbered that from South to North for almost a decade), from countries such as Egypt, Lebanon or Jordan to Gulf countries (e.g., Saudi Arabia, Oman, Kuwait, Bahrain, and the United Arab Emirates), or from Venezuela to Colombia, Brazil, or Ecuador. These migrant workers are also excluded from the social security system, and the pandemic further exacerbated their already uncertain socio-economic situation. In Gulf countries, as in Canada, irregular migrants have limited access to healthcare while living "in conditions that facilitate the transmission of the virus (dwellings, dormitories or camps, where maintaining a social distance is difficult and access to water and hygiene infrastructure is limited)" (Mabille 2021, 26). Venezuelans face high unemployment in the Latin

American countries that have taken them in, and they were hit disproportionately by wage cuts during the pandemic (Chaves-González et al. 2021). There is a lack of migrant worker and refugee integration into host societies here and elsewhere.

International Students

Student mobility has been on the rise worldwide since the early 1990s. According to the Migration Data Portal, some 3.3 million of a total of 5.3 million international students (enrolled in graduate programmes) in 2017 chose North America and Europe as their host destination. These students were affected by pandemic restrictions, including isolation from campus closures and the loss of their student jobs.

Student mobility—which is more or less accessible depending on the political context and an individual's socioeconomic situation—is not always synonymous with upward social mobility. Often considered to fall somewhere between migrant and tourist, these "citizens of the world" whose talents, good fortune, and bright futures are internationally celebrated are more often than not seen as part of an elite (see literature review in Sanchez 2020; Waters 2012). In a way, the COVID-19 pandemic highlighted their precarity, particularly in North America. In spring 2020, international students once again became "migrants like any others," because of their vulnerability when what they came to do—i.e., study—could not be done under the usual conditions. A very large number of them now associate the pandemic with a real-world example of sudden precarity.

Like agricultural and healthcare workers, international students play a crucial role in the economy. In Canada, international student tuition is much higher than that for Canadian students, and some universities' profits depend on these cohorts, as their tuition partly reduces the gap between operating expenses (which are increasing) and provincial grants (which are stagnating). In 2017–2018, nearly one third of mathematics, computer, and information science students enrolled in Canadian universities came from abroad. Because this population also constitutes an expected specialized workforce, the pandemic-induced immobilization of international students will impact university finances and economic recovery. International students are also a major driver for the recreation and tourism industry.

In the United States and Canada, this perception of international students as a source of income stands in stark contrast to the way in which the government's pandemic assistance measures remained largely—if not fully—inaccessible to them. In the United States, international students (one million by spring 2020) are still not eligible for federal aid, and their right to work is limited to campuses. In Quebec, the 20-hour-per-week restriction on international students' right to work has been relaxed. However, international students were not eligible for the Canada Emergency Student Benefit (CESB), as it was for citizens and permanent residents only. Many of them were also ineligible for the CERB, as they did not always meet the previous income criteria.

As the various impacts of the pandemic and related health measures emerged, the North American media reported on the psychological distress international students experienced from the rapid deterioration of their living conditions (e.g., housing, food, allowances, and mobility). The rapid and sudden closure of student residences—both in the United States and Canada—was widely reported. An accumulation of negative impacts hit some students hardest, such as those whose income was guaranteed by university funding (grants) or whose continued presence on campus in fall 2020 was conditional on their being there, despite the health risks (e.g., at Boston College).

Where farm workers lack organized support, student associations have helped alert and mobilize the public about residential housing and administrative issues (visas and permits). The Canadian authorities granted a number of concessions concerning the right of temporary residence, for example, the request to extend study permits until 31 December 2020—initially rejected—was then approved, with implied status, and the automatic renewal of rights for students whose applications had been validated before 19 March 2020. In the United States, the Department of Homeland Security allowed international students (F-1 visa) to retain their status in the country even if they were doing their studies online—from within the United States or abroad.

What's Next?

Since March 2020, migrant workers have been at the front lines of the pandemic response. The COVID-19 pandemic exacerbated and highlighted the precarity they face, becoming a well-documented public issue that widespread media coverage brought out of the shadows. More often than not, crises reinforce—rather than subvert—migration trends (Geddes 2021). Can the pandemic reverse this trend? The pandemic could be a key opportunity to introduce public policies and mechanisms (in addition to the temporary easing of several measures [for OECD countries, see OECD 2020]) that would enable migrants to express themselves and be subject to the law like any other worker.

The solutions to most of these precarious situations are well known. For example, the Global Compact for Migration (2018) provides for the essentials of a systemic program to "standardize" immigration in our societies. It would take time to implement and action to encourage governments to draw inspiration from it. It remains to be seen whether the current crisis will have any real effect on public preferences—in the long term—for different types of migrant workers, particularly those in so-called "essential" jobs. The pandemic has also shown that, in times of crisis, barriers to migration are more easily surmountable. For example, the easing of restrictions on foreign-trained healthcare workers; an appeal to refugee doctors with no recognized qualifications in Germany; and the accelerated recognition of such qualifications in the United Kingdom.

The pandemic also allowed more people to see and understand the precarious status and—consequently—social conditions of too many migrant workers. Lifting this labour market out of the exploitative bubble in which it is trapped, or funding universities using different budgetary methods (one of the recommendations of the Royal Society of Canada's 2021 briefing) are above all political decisions.

Remedying this situation requires giving migrant workers a "voice" and the ability to defend their rights. They must be able to report abuses to credible institutions (e.g., Human Rights Commission, grievance arbitrators, or tribunals), without fear of reprisals from employers or of being deported from the country. Workers in the sectors mentioned—migrants or not—must be able to associate, unionize, and negotiate their working conditions just like many other workers do.

Labour laws must also be applied consistently. In particular, workplace inspections must be able to focus their attention on all economic sectors where precarity gives rise to exploitation. To achieve this, migrant workers' precarious immigration status must be eliminated, which involves scrapping single-employer work permits and giving these workers access to automatically renewable work permits of at least one year, followed by permanent residency. All requests to normalize abnormal situations must be reviewed rapidly, with a priority on stabilizing the status of these workers. In addition, all residents of a country, whatever their status—or lack of status—must have access to essential benefits.

The light the pandemic shed on our economies could provide an opportunity to engage in an in-depth conversation with the public about the important role immigration plays in our economic, social, and political progress, to change people's mindsets. A post-pandemic world centred on rebuilding will need to be coupled with political reflection on the social improvement of its most vulnerable.

Notes

1.   Ontario(AttorneyGeneral)v.Fraser,2011SCC20[2011]2S.C.R.3,seehttps://scc-csc. lexum.com/scc-csc/scc-csc/en/item/7934/index.do.

References

Bassi, Marie, and Farida Souiah. 2019. "La violence du régime des frontières et ses conséquences létales : récits et pratiques autour des morts et disparus par migration." *Critique internationale* 2, no. 83 (May): 9–19.

Boucher, Anna, and Justin Gest. 2018. *Crossroads: Comparative Immigration Regimes in a World of Demographic Change.* New York: Cambridge University Press.

Butler, Judith. 2009. *Frames of War: When Is Life Grievable?* London: Verso.

Chaves-González, Diego, Jordi Amaral, and María Jesús Mora. 2021. *Socioeconomic Integration of Venezuelan Migrants and Refugees. The Cases of Brazil, Chile, Colombia, Ecuador, and Peru.* IOM UN Migration and MPI (Migration Policy Institute) Report, July 2021. https://www.iom. int/sites/g/files/tmzbdl486/files/press_release/file/mpi-iom_socioeconomic-integration-venezuelans_2021_final.pdf.

Dauvergne, Catherine. 2016. *The New Politics of Immigration and the End of Settler Societies.* New York: Cambridge University Press.

Geddes, Andrew. 2021. "Objective and Subjective Migration Trends in Europe." *Migration Policy Practice* 11, no. 1 (January–February).

ILO (International Labour Organization). 2018. "Estimations mondiales de l'OIT concernant les travailleuses et les travailleurs migrants : résultats et méthodologie : résumé", Department of Statistics, 2nd edition, Geneva: BIT.

IOM (International Organization for Migration). 2021. *Global Migration Restriction Overview.* https://migration.iom.int/reports/covid-19-travel-restrictions-output-%E2%80%94-22-march-2021.

Mabille, Claire, 2021. "Les migrations à l'épreuve d'une pandémie." *Revue défense nationale.* HS3, special issue: 25–30.

Migration Data Portal. 2023. "Migration Data Relevant for the COVID-19 Pandemic." https://www.migrationdataportal.org/themes/migration-data-relevant-covid-19-pandemic.

OECD (Organisation for Economic Co-operation and Development). 2019. *Recent Trends in International Migration of Doctors, Nurses and Medical Students*. Paris: OECD Publishing. https://www.oecd-ilibrary.org/sites/5571ef48-en/index.html?itemId=/content/publication/5571ef48-en.

———. 2020. "Contribution of Migrant Doctors and Nurses to Tackling COVID-19 Crisis in OECD Countries." *Tackling Coronavirus Brief*, May 13, 2020. Paris: OECD Publishing. https://read.oecd-ilibrary.org/view/?ref=132_132856-kmg6jh3kvd&title=Contribution-of-migrant-doctors-and-nurses-to-tackling-COVID-19-crisis-in-OECD-countries.

Pew Research Centre. 2020. "More than Nine-in-Ten People Worldwide Live in Countries with Travel Restrictions amid COVID-19." https://www.pewresearch.org/fact-tank/2020/04/01/more-than-nine-in-ten-people-worldwide-live-in-countries-with-travel-restrictions-amid-covid-19/.

Sanchez, Inès. 2020. "Trajectoires d'étudiants français à McGill et HEC Montréal. Une reproduction sociale et culturelle en mobilité." Master's thesis, International Studies, Université de Montréal.

United Nations General Assembly. 2018. *Global Compact for Safe, Orderly and Regular Migration*. Final document of the Intergovernmental Conference to Adopt the Global Compact for Safe, Orderly and Regular Migration. December 10 to 11, 2018. https://www.ohchr.org/en/migration/global-compact-safe-orderly-and-regular-migration-gcmHO

Waters, Johanna L. 2012. "Geographies of International Education: Mobilities and the Reproduction of Social (Dis)advantage." *Geography Compass* 6, no. 3 (March): 123–136.

World Health Organization. 2010. *WHO Global Code of Practice on the International Recruitment of Health Personnel*. https://www.who.int/publications/i/item/wha68.32.

Wilson, Thomas M., and Hastings Donnan, eds. 2012. *A Companion to Border Studies*. Oxford: John Wiley & Sons.

Conclusion

Jennifer Welsh and Frédéric Mérand

We wrote the first draft of these concluding pages in the final days of 2021, during a week in which several countries reimposed stringent travel rules and tightened social restrictions in the face of another mutation of COVID-19—the Omicron variant. This deadly chapter in the story of the pandemic showed us that, while COVID-19 arrived and spread across the world with great speed, its ending would be much more difficult to determine and declare. If, when, and how we entered the "post-pandemic" world are thus questions that continue to preoccupy scientists and policy makers to this day.

In the months before the first wave of Omicron, various countries—and constituencies within countries—were experimenting with life after COVID-19. Mask mandates were being loosened and hand sanitizer was no longer a scarce commodity. Some employees were beginning to return to their workplaces and universities were resuming many of their in-person classes. Governments were announcing phase-outs of their emergency subsidies and special pandemic programs. And in many parts of the world, families and individuals were making plans to spend the holidays, in person, with their loved ones.

Many of these plans were, of course, derailed by the emergence of the Omicron variant, which reminded us that living with various versions of COVID-19 is now part of our reality. In the time since this conclusion was written, COVID-19 has become endemic, and will continue to be at least for the immediate future. However, despite the prolongation of our collective ride on this rollercoaster, it is still possible to offer observations about how we—in Canada and in the world—confronted a once-in-a-generation challenge.

Challenging Dominant Narratives

The onset and evolution of COVID-19 generated many definitive and sweeping judgments. We were told early on, for example, that autocratic states were better prepared and better structured to tackle a public health emergency, given their capacities for efficiency and control, whereas democracies were limited in their abilities to produce and enforce effective public policy. We witnessed economic analysts wringing their hands about record-high debt levels, which they predicted would constrain future policy making. We heard frequent laments about the failure of international cooperation—and of particular intergovernmental institutions—to confront a common health threat. And we faced apocalyptic warnings about an inevitable cold war between the U.S. and China, which the pandemic had clearly accelerated and deepened.

Lurking beneath these larger structural forces, however, is another story about the pandemic. It is a story of micro-level variation rather than broad patterns; of small wins rather than big failures; and of "islands of cooperation" rather than wholescale strategic rivalry.

A Task for Future Social Scientists? Explaining Variation

The pandemic was not good for democracy. In 2020, the Economist Intelligence Unit's Democracy Index reached its lowest point since 2006, as governments used emergency measures to prevent mobility (in democracies) or stifle protest and dissent (elsewhere) (Economist Intelligence Unit 2020). Some governments, like that of Thailand, turned fully authoritarian; others, like that of Brazil, used illiberal discourse to deflect public attention from the leader's mismanagement of the COVID-19 crisis. In most democracies, most notably the United States, public health measures emboldened an anti-lockdown and anti-vaccine movement, which has merged with pre-existing populist parties to create a potent anti-system force. And yet, at least in European countries in the short term, preliminary data showed that support for incumbent governments and trust in political institutions actually increased during the pandemic, suggesting that there was a positive "rally-around-the-flag" effect when people needed help and turned to government (Bol et al. 2021). In Canada, the 2021 election was more ambiguous: despite early indications that the Trudeau government might win a majority on the back of its efforts to protect and support Canadians during COVID-19, the composition of the House of Commons looked remarkably similar to its pre-election version after the votes were counted.

That said, no political system had (or has) a monopoly on best practice in pandemic preparedness and response. Some of the world's successful democracies performed reasonably well in tackling COVID-19; others—including, at various times in the first two years of the pandemic, the United States—fared spectacularly badly. Countries like Sweden were alternately hailed as culturally more resilient and lambasted as politically insensitive. The performance of the world's largest democracy, India, was all over the map. After a deadly first wave and harsh lockdown, government officials were declaring the "endgame" in the first quarter of 2021 (*The Lancet* 2021), as the country appeared, on the surface, to be weathering the virus better than others. By May 2021, however, India was responsible for more than half of the world's coronavirus daily case counts, setting records of close to 400,000 cases per day. Overall, the country stands as a study in contradictions: though it is one of the world's leading vaccine manufacturers, as of late November 2021 it had fully vaccinated only 3 percent of its population (*The New York Times* 2021).

For years to come, social scientists will be searching for the particular conditions—political, social, economic, geographic, and cultural—that explain why, when faced with the same virus, societies adopted different approaches to addressing COVID-19 with varying degrees of success, not only in minimizing infections and deaths but also in "Building Back Better." Given that the pandemic was a "total social fact," to borrow, as we did in the introduction, from French sociologist Marcel Mauss, these explanations are unlikely to be monocausal. Nor will they always rely on deeper structural factors; the specific features of national character and the impacts of individual political leadership, both positive and negative, will also be part of the mix. What is likely to emerge is an account in which prior vulnerabilities—whether social, economic, or institutional—were laid bare by the onslaught of a deadly virus. Perhaps we will also see greater appreciation of the role of political judgement in times of great urgency.

Rewriting the Fiscal Rulebook

It is also difficult to make definitive judgments about the audacity of the fiscal policies adopted during the eye of the COVID-19 storm. What is certain is that the capacity of rich-world governments to plug holes in the economy has proved greater than hitherto imagined. Between March 2020 and March 2021, massive stimulus and recovery programs were adopted in the U.S., in the EU, and in Canada: additional budget spending reached $20 trillion, or 16 percent of global domestic product. Low interest rates and an evolving economic paradigm shaped by the experience of the Great Recession propelled North American and European governments to roll out the largest economic stimulus packages yet seen in peacetime. In doing so, they seem to have learned from the lessons of the 2008 financial and economic crisis, when public spending was too late, too modest, and withdrawn too quickly.

Unbeknownst to most of us at the time, central banks around the world coordinated a multi-billion-dollar injection of liquidity to ensure financial stability during the first days of the Great Lockdown. They then continued the quantitative easing measures tested during the previous recession, buying treasury bonds so that governments could spend almost without limit and keeping interest rates low to keep the economy churning. Thanks to these measures, governments like that of Canada were able to implement vigorous income support measures that not only helped prevent industrial and social collapse but also led to an impressive economic rebound the year after lockdown (Tooze 2021). Despite historic public deficits, ballooning government debt, and fears of long-term inflation, most rich countries were back to pre-pandemic economic figures by 2021. This result seemed to justify the decision made by most governments to violate the norm of low deficits that had been commonplace since the 1990s.

This daring fiscal response was a small policy win that averted a big economic and social failure. It led to hopes that the COVID-19 crisis might become an opportunity for a "Great Reset," to use the theme of the postponed 2021 World Economic Forum at Davos. These hopes were soon dashed, however, and the long-term picture now seems less rosy. With NextGenerationEU, European leaders adopted the largest coordinated recovery program in their common history, involving real cash transfers to afflicted Member States and joint borrowing. It is too early to tell if this strategy will shift the institutional nature and culture of the EU towards permanent solidarity. In the United States, Joe Biden won the presidential election with the slogan "Build Back Better," promising to create a European-style welfare state with higher environmental ambitions, but he was forced to back down in the face of Senate opposition (Joanis, Mérand, and Bezzaz 2021). Everywhere, mounting government debt and rising inflation will make a second Keynesian response, in the event of a prolonged economic crisis or another lockdown, much more difficult to implement.

By contrast, emerging markets and developing countries accumulated record public debt, even though they spent much less on recovery than rich countries (Gaspar, Medas, and Perrelli 2021). What is noteworthy is how the World Bank and other large creditors stepped up to the plate with a $93 billion support package (World Bank 2021). This is another example of remarkable coordination within international financial institutions flying in the face of a presumed national egoism. This also shows that international technocracies can learn lessons from past crises. But like the COVAX mechanism, which was marred by delays and unfulfilled promises (see below), it is not clear how much money will ultimately be disbursed to the benefit of fiscally constrained governments. There is also a limit to the extent to which governments can shape the perceptions of financial markets. As interest rates rise, public debt will cripple poor countries for years to come, as these countries never had the same amount of fiscal slack as rich ones in the first place.

Rethinking Cooperation

As suggested above, the story of cooperation during the pandemic is more complex than the standard condemnation of the ways in which national governments turned inward rather than outward in search of solutions to the pandemic.

On the one hand, it is undeniable that, for much of the first two years of the pandemic, states failed to work effectively through international institutions to harmonize public health policies, share burdens, and reach reciprocal agreements. Instead, governments engaged in forms of global policy *competition* through a race for scarce resources and "beggar-thy-neighbour" strategies. Where state interaction did occur, it largely took the form of *ad hoc* policy-borrowing, or emulation, from jurisdictions that seemed to be addressing the pandemic successfully, rather than a conscious effort to coordinate. Some leaders also indulged in the well-worn tradition of scapegoating international institutions (most notably the WHO) and diverting attention from the failures of their own national policies.

As a result, state behaviour fell far short of what the academic literature identifies as core requirements for effective action on transnational threats such as infectious disease: far-sighted collaboration that aims for long-term solutions to shared threats, a degree of deference to experts with specialized knowledge, and multilateral cooperation through international institutions (Johnson 2020). The May 2021 Global Health Summit of the G20—the first meeting of its kind—offered heads of state what some have called their "San Francisco moment" for setting clear goals and initiating bold collective action on pandemic preparedness and response (Bose and Pillary 2021). However, while the final declaration did acknowledge the need for stronger and sustained support for multilateral cooperation, it only went as far as to elaborate a set of guiding principles to improve collective action on pandemics and other broader global health objectives and emphasized the "voluntary orientation" of state commitments.[1] No specific targets, actions, or timeframes were set out. The meeting of G7 leaders that followed in mid-June of 2021 did generate more ambitious pledges to "vaccinate the world" (through both the donation of vaccines and increased funding for distribution), as well as calls to improve global surveillance of infectious disease and support the WHO.[2] Nevertheless, even on the high-visibility issue of vaccines, G7 promises of 870 million doses fell far short of the 11 billion doses estimated to be essential to ensure 70 percent of the world's population is vaccinated against COVID-19 by the end of 2022.

If the key ingredients for effective cooperation were in short supply to face the common pandemic threat, they were even more scarce with respect to simmering conflicts and instability. The call of the Secretary-General of the UN for a "global ceasefire" in the spring of 2020 gained very little traction, both among combatants and key states with the diplomatic influence to shape conflict trajectories. After a short-lived "calming down" effect of the pandemic on political violence, the security situation deteriorated in many parts of the world, from Ethiopia, where civil war erupted in November 2020; to the Sahel, where French, African, and UN forces failed to contain jihadist expansion. The conflict in Afghanistan reached a tipping point in the summer of 2021 when the Taliban looked set to take Kabul, prompting a hasty and humiliating Western withdrawal as well as a humanitarian catastrophe that continues to unfold.

The high point of the return of interstate conflict is in Ukraine, which was brutally invaded by Russia in February 2022. For many observers, the liberal international order that was put in place after the end of the Cold War in 1989 was buried by the pandemic and the return of war in Europe. Meanwhile, tensions increased between the United States and China over Taiwan and the South China Sea. The fact that the United States was widely seen as having lost its ability to impose global order, while all the international attention was focused on the pandemic, may help to explain why relations were further deteriorating between the world's two superpowers.

Underneath the lacklustre performance of states and intergovernmental institutions, however, was an alternative form of cooperation on a micro scale. From the earliest moments of the detection of the virus, scientific communities moved rapidly to share data and genetic sequences and pharmaceutical companies worked feverishly to develop COVID-19 vaccines, thereby illustrating the power of transnational collaboration *below* the state level.[3] The speed and geographic spread of those working on vaccines and other medical countermeasures was both impressive and unprecedented. Much of this effort took place *without* formal state-to-state coordination, either bilaterally or in international organizations. Technology played a major part in this story, enabling collaborative research, findings, and vaccines to circulate more quickly and globally than ever before among individuals, scientists, firms, and authorities.

Another example of cooperative action was the launch in April 2020 of the Access to COVID-19 Tools (ACT) Accelerator. Hosted by the WHO, this mechanism convened scientists, governments, business, civil society, philanthropists, and global health organizations to accelerate the development of tests, treatments, and vaccines, and to ensure their equal distribution. The vaccine pillar of the ACT Accelerator, COVAX, was designed to function as a central procurement mechanism for all countries wherein wealthier countries would buy into the scheme and their funding would finance COVID-19 vaccines for low-income countries. COVAX was thus intended to operationalize the idea of global solidarity by ensuring that all countries, including low- and middle-income ones, would receive a share of the vaccines purchased. While in practice COVAX had a mixed record, suggesting the need for a more ambitious and permanent platform to ensure equitable access to vital tests, treatments, and vaccines in future pandemics,[4] it remains a positive example of the kind of multistakeholder cooperation needed to tackle common global challenges.

Finding "Islands of Agreement"

In her fascinating study of interstate rivalries between Israel and Lebanon, India and Pakistan, and Greece and Turkey, Gabriella Blum (2007) argues that even within the most entrenched and bitter conflicts, adversaries can carve out limited areas that remain safe or even prosperous amid a tide of war. As her work shows, these havens of cooperative exchange effectively reduce competition and loss, allowing mutually beneficial exchanges to take place and offering hope for broader accords in the future.

The same could be said of the interactions between China and the United States over the initial years of the pandemic. This is not to underplay the degree of geopolitical competition that marked the behaviour of the two superpowers, including in their approach to the public health emergency and particularly in the realm of vaccines. As noted in the introduction, China adroitly stepped into the global vaccine access crisis by selling and donating vaccines in ways that advanced its foreign policy interests, with doses primarily going to states participating in its Belt and Road Initiative. In turn, worries about China (and to a lesser extent Russia) gaining a "first mover advantage" in assisting strategically important countries led the United States to engage in its own form of vaccine diplomacy through the vaccine initiative, launched by the Quadrilateral Security Dialogue in March 2021, and the decisions reached on vaccine sharing at the G7 meeting in June 2021. At the Global COVID-19 Summit he convened in the autumn of 2021, President Biden coupled his pledge of an additional 500 million Pfizer doses with the claim that the United States was now the world's "arsenal of vaccines," thereby invoking his country's role in the Second World War and revealing the political motives underpinning its global health policy.

But China and the United States have also shared certain interests and perspectives. One example is their lukewarm response to ongoing negotiations for a new legal instrument to strengthen the world's system for pandemic preparedness and response.[5] Washington's position on a so-called pandemic treaty has been particularly disappointing to EU states, who have been the drivers of this initiative, but so too has the diplomatic stance of Beijing. Both states have also refrained from backing calls for an enhancement of the powers of the WHO—for example, to conduct more effective investigations of "disease events"—or for an increase in assessed contributions to the organization. Indeed, while the United States under President Biden has been lauded for its "return" to the WHO, its behaviour in both the past and present does not indicate that Washington necessarily prioritizes this intergovernmental forum for the realization of its global health priorities. It is worth remembering that previous signature initiatives by the United States in global health, such as the 2003 President's Emergency Plan for AIDS Relief, was a bilateral rather than multilateral initiative and stemmed in large part from concerns that the disease could destabilize countries in the region, enabling transnational and criminal organizations to use African territories as a base from which to harm the United States (Fidler 2021). It appears, then, that both the United States and China approach global health less through the lens of securing the supply of a global public good and more through the lens of advancing key geostrategic interests.

The other key interest shared by these two states is climate change. On this front, the EU has led the way with the adoption of the most ambitious and credible greenhouse gas emission reductions targets. But a public good like climate can only be tackled through a joint effort between the world's two biggest emitters, China and the United States (Froggat and Quiggin 2021). It is good news, therefore, that the Chinese Communist Party and U.S. Democrats see eye to eye on the need to reach carbon neutrality—by 2060 for China and 2050 for the United States Although these countries are economic competitors with massive carbon footprints, both face the same domestic and international pressures to reduce emissions. Climate change thus remains a likely arena for micro-cooperation between Beijing and Washington: no matter how warm or cold Sino–American relations are, the green energy transition they are both invested in relies on minerals, material, technology, and supply chains that are complementary and indeed intertwined at the global level (Meao 2021).

Assessing the Damage: Legacies of Inequality

While our analysis calls into question some of the stories we have been told about COVID-19, there is one central plot line that resonates with all the contributors to this book: the story of how the pandemic illustrated and heightened inequality among and within societies. In some cases, the disparities have been glaring, as with the persistent inequity in vaccine coverage: at the end of 2021, 73 percent of all COVID-19 vaccines administered globally were to the citizens of high- and upper-middle-income countries, with only 0.8 percent to those of low-income countries.[6] This stark disparity was one of the main explanations for why new variants were able to emerge and spread throughout the world.

In other cases, the disparities have been more subtle and insidious. Analysis by the World Bank indicates that, while all countries have experienced negative economic consequences as a result of the pandemic, some have clearly been hit harder than others. Prior to COVID-19, average incomes across countries had been converging, with inequality between countries falling by 34 percent between 1993 and 2017 (World Bank 2016), but the pandemic appeared to have reversed this trend. The figures for 2017 to 2021 revealed a 1.2 percent growth in between-country inequality—the first increase in a generation (Yonzan, Lakner, and Gerszon Mahler 2021). Governments that have emerged exhausted and heavily indebted from the Great Lockdown, or whose GDP depended to a large extent on remittances from their impoverished diaspora, will have limited access to credit and less capacity to provide basic services or build public infrastructure for their populations. Notwithstanding China and a few other exceptions, the catching-up process that began in earnest in the early 2000s will decelerate or stop altogether as the gap between the Global South and rich countries widens once more.

Rising income inequality also operates at the micro level. Using the same methodology that the World Bank applies to the study of global poverty, analysis of recent data shows a significant divergence between richer and poorer parts of the global income distribution. In 2021, the richest two deciles were expected to recover nearly half of their 2020 losses on average, while the poorest two deciles were expected to lose a further 5 percent of their income on average.[7] As the *New York Times* reported one year after the onset of the spring 2020 global lockdown, any initial hopes that the pandemic might be a "great equalizer" were quickly overshadowed by the realities of a great divide in COVID-19 outcomes, based upon class, race, and gender (Serkez 2021). The effects of the virus in the United States—whether economic or medical—varied significantly depending on whether you were an essential worker or could work from home during the height of the pandemic, or whether you became unemployed, thus suffering both drastic declines in income and worrying levels of food insecurity. To fully comprehend the inequities of the pandemic, one needs to look beyond national frontiers to examine the fate of specific subnational groups.

Once we do so, the distinctions between wealthy and poor countries begin to fade. José Alvarez's fascinating analysis of the United States, Brazil, and India (three countries that were heavily affected by the pandemic) demonstrates that structural inequalities and pre-existing socioeconomic vulnerabilities, combined with specific government policies adopted during the pandemic, underpinned the unequal effects of COVID-19 on particular pockets of the population. These included Black, Latinx, and Indigenous communities in the United States, individuals identified by pigmentation or indigenous origins in Brazil, and persons defined by caste in India. Notwithstanding striking differences in GDP, Alvarez finds that, across all three countries, groups long disadvantaged by neo-colonialist legacies associated with race, ethnicity, or social status have endured COVID-19's harshest effects, from infection to hospitalization to death (Alvarez 2022). His preliminary data on other parts of the world reveal similar trends across Latin America and Africa, where poverty levels alone cannot account for disproportionate health outcomes related to the pandemic. In short, there appears to be a COVID "colour line" crossing the globe, revealing stark racial, ethnic, and other social divides.

In this global picture, Canada has fared better. Although the pandemic also exposed structural inequalities and vulnerabilities in our country, with low-income women and visible minorities more likely to catch the disease or lose their jobs, unprecedented government transfers have led to a growth in disposable income and wealth for the lowest-income households. At least in the short term, COVID-19 has led to a reduction in economic inequality in Canada (Statistics Canada 2021). While this trend may very well be reversed as fiscal consolidation takes hold, the Canadian experience shows the difference that progressive and pragmatic policy solutions can make in times of crisis.

The Elusive "Afterworld"

In convening the contributors to this project, we intended to tap into the reservoir of hope that seemed to be accumulating about the possibility of "Building Back Better" after the pandemic. The spring of 2020 was a time in which many dared to dream about the positive transformations that might emerge from the devastation of COVID-19. And yet, as we have observed at various points in this book, crises are not, in and of themselves, capable of producing progressive change.

They only present the *possibility* of change. As we produced this book, we observed instead a palpable longing in many corners to "get back to normal" — to life *before* the pandemic.

This longing begs the question of what "normal" now means. If we accept the argument that COVID-19 has been more a moment of great revelation than one of profound rupture, we might expect the troubling trends exposed by the virus — democratic recession, growing inequality, accelerating climate change, and runaway technological development — to continue to affect the shape and certainty of the world we once knew. In this context, the search for normal is likely to be an elusive one. Rather than confronting an "Afterworld," societies will be grappling with an economic, social, and political "long COVID," which will transform our pre-pandemic existence into a quaint memory.

Notes

1. The concluding statement of the summit, the Rome Declaration, is available at https://global-health-summit.europa.eu/rome-declaration_en.
2. See the Carbis Bay G7 Summit Communiqué, June 13, 2021. Available at https://www.whitehouse.gov/briefing-room/statements-releases/2021/06/13/carbis-bay-g7-summit-communique/.
3. This "below the state" cooperation was of various kinds, including collaboration among scientists (through the Coalition for Epidemic Preparedness Innovations), among different pharmaceutical companies (Pfizer working alongside BioNTech), and between scientific communities and private companies (AstraZeneca collaborating with the University of Oxford).
4. This is one of the key proposals of the Independent Panel created by the WHO to review the response to COVID-19. See *COVID-19: Make It the Last Pandemic*, Report of the Independent Panel on Pandemic Preparedness and Response, May 12, 2021. Available at https://theindependentpanel.org/wp-content/uploads/2021/05/COVID-19-Make-it-the-Last-Pandemic_final.pdf. The proposals of the Independent Panel, which envisage "end-to-end" planning for research and development, technology transfer, clinical trials, and manufacturing processes, are designed to transform pandemic preparedness and response from a charity model to a shared-fate model, in which more societies participate in the production and distribution of the requirements for meeting potential pandemic challenges.
5. The Special Session of the World Health Assembly in November 2021 agreed to begin negotiations on a new "instrument" or "accord" to better govern pandemic preparedness and response. While the framework convention under discussion is being referred to as a "pandemic treaty," Member States have not converged on the idea of a legally binding treaty. For further discussion, see "Q and A: After the World Health Assembly Special Session, How Likely Is a Pandemic Treaty?," *United Nations Foundation*, December 6, 2021. Available at https://unfoundation.org/blog/post/qa-after-the-world-health-assembly-special-session-how-likely-is-a-pandemic-treaty/.
6. See the Covid World Vaccination Tracker. Available at https://www.nytimes.com/interactive/2021/world/covid-vaccinations-tracker.html.

7.   See Yonzan, Lakner, and Gerszon Mahler 2021. This divergence holds even when individuals in China and India are excluded from the global sample.

References

Alvarez, José E. 2022. "The Case for Reparations for the Color of COVID." *UCI Journal of International, Transnational and Comparative Law 7*.

Blum, Gabriella. 2007. *Islands of Agreement: Managing Enduring Armed Rivalries.* Cambridge: Harvard University Press.

Bol, Damien, Marco Giani, André Blais, and Peter J. Loewen. 2021. "The Effect of COVID-19 Lockdowns on Political Support: Some Good News for Democracy?" *European Journal of Political Research* 60, no. 2 (May): 497–505.

Bose, Kent, and Yogan Pillary. 2021. "The 2021 Rome Global Health Summit: A Missed Opportunity." *BMJ Opinion*, May 25, 2021. https://blogs.bmj.com/bmj/2021/05/25/the-2021-rome-global-health-summit-a-missed-opportunity/.

Economist Intelligence Unit. 2020. *Democracy Index 2020: In Sickness and in Health?* London: Economic Intelligence Unit. https://www.eiu.com/n/campaigns/democracy-index-2020/.

Fidler, David P. 2021. "A New Era in U.S. Global Health Leadership? What the World Health Assembly Meeting Revealed." Think Global Health, June 3, 2021. https://www.thinkglobalhealth.org/article/new-era-us-global-health-leadership.

Froggat, Antony, and Daniel Quiggin. 2021. "China, EU and US Cooperation on Climate and Energy: An Ever-Changing Relationship." Research Report. London: Chatham House.

Gaspar, Vitor, Paulo Medas, and Roberto Perrelli. 2021. "Global Debt Reaches a Record $226 Trillion." *IMF Blog*, December 15, 2021. https://blogs.imf.org/2021/12/15/global-debt-reaches-a-record-226-trillion/.

Joanis, Marcelin, Frédéric Mérand, and Meryem Bezzaz. 2021. *L'effet COVID: la relance économique et l'investissement public en perspective comparée.* Cahiers du CÉRIUM 26.

Johnson, Tana. 2020. "Ordinary Patterns in an Extraordinary Crisis: How International Relations Makes Sense of the COVID-19 Pandemic." *International Organization*, 74(S1): E148–E168.

The Lancet. 2021. "India's COVID-19 Emergency." *The Lancet* 397, no. 1683 (May): 1683. https://www.thelancet.com/journals/lancet/article/PIIS0140-6736(21)01052-7/fulltext.

Meao, Paul. 2021. "Can China and the United States Cooperate Fully in Tackling Climate Change?," *The Diplomat*, November 1, 2021. https://thediplomat.com/2021/11/can-china-and-the-united-states-cooperate-fully-in-tackling-climate-change/.

The New York Times. 2021. "What to Know about India's Coronavirus Crisis." *The New York Times,* November 17, 2021. https://www.nytimes.com/article/india-coronavirus-cases-deaths.html.

Serkez, Yaryna. "These Charts Show that Your Lockdown Experience Wasn't Just about Luck." *The New York Times,* March 14, 2021. https://www.nytimes.com/interactive/2021/03/11/opinion/covid-inequality-race-gender.html.

Statistics Canada. 2021. "Household Economic Well-Being during the COVID-19 Pandemic, Experimental Estimates, First Quarter to Third Quarter of 2020." Statistics Canada, March 1, 2021. https://www150.statcan.gc.ca/n1/daily-quotidien/210301/dq210301b-eng.htm.

Tooze, Adam. 2021. *Shutdown: How Covid Shook the World's Economy.* New York: Penguin.

World Bank 2016. *Poverty and Shared Prosperity 2016: Take on Inequality.* Washington, D.C.: World Bank. https://openknowledge.worldbank.org/bitstream/handle/10986/25078/9781464809583.pdf?sequence=24&isAllowed=y.

——. 2021. "Global Community Steps Up with $93 Billion Support Package to Boost Resilient Recovery in World's Poorest Countries." Press release, December 15, 2021. https://www.worldbank.org/en/news/press-release/2021/12/15/global-community-steps-up-with-93-billion-support-package-to-boost-resilient-recovery-in-world-s-poorest-countries.

Yonzan, Nishant, Christopher Lakner, and Daniel Gerszon Mahler. 2021. "Is COVID-19 Increasing Global Inequality?" *World Bank Blogs,* October 7, 2021. https://blogs.worldbank.org/opendata/covid-19-increasing-global-inequality.

List of Contributors

Anthony Amicelle, Université de Montréal
Valérie Amiraux, Université de Montréal
Vincent Arel-Bundock, Université de Montréal
Ari Van Assche, HEC Montréal
Daniel Béland, McGill University
Karim Benyekhlef, Université de Montréal
Mark R. Brawley, McGill University
Dominique Caouette, Université de Montréal
Allison Christians, McGill University
Ryoa Chung, Université de Montréal
François Crépeau, McGill University
Pierre-Marie David, Université de Montréal
Magdalena Dembińska, Université de Montréal
Peter Dietsch, Université de Montréal
Thomas Druetz, Université de Montréal
Pearl Eliadis, McGill University
Philippe Fournier, Collège Brébeuf
François Furstenberg, Johns-Hopkins University
Alain Gagnon, Université de Montréal
Pablo Gilabert, Concordia University
Timothy Hodges, McGill University
Maya Jegen, Université du Québec à Montréal
Juliet Johnson, McGill University

Nicholas King, McGill University
Erick Lachapelle, Université de Montréal
Sonia Laszlo, McGill University
Justin Leroux, HEC Montréal
Pierre Martin, Université de Montréal
Sarah-Myriam Martin-Brûlé, Bishops University
María Martín de Almagro Iniesta, Université de Montréal
Erik Martinez Kuhonta, McGill University
Theodore McLauchlin, Université de Montréal
Frédéric Mégret, McGill University
Frédéric Mérand, Université de Montréal
Cynthia Milton, University of Victoria
Laurence Monnais, Université de Montréal
Christian Novak, McGill University
Mireille Paquet, Concordia University
T.V. Paul, McGill University
Krzysztof Pelc, McGill University
Pierre-Olivier Pineau, HEC Montréal
Vincent Pouliot, McGill University
René Provost, McGill University
Lee Seymour, Université de Montréal
Thomas Soehl, McGill University
Maïka Sondarjee, University of Ottawa
Samuel Tanner, Université de Montréal
Jean-Philippe Thérien, Université de Montréal
Hamish van der Ven, University of British Columbia
Luna Vives, Université de Montréal
Jennifer Welsh, McGill University
Marie-Joëlle Zahar, Université de Montréal

Health and Society

Health occupies a central place in public debate, and the *Health and Society* series provides a space for dialogue on different fields of expertise (sociology, psychology, political science, biology, nutrition, medicine, nursing, human kinetics, and rehabilitation sciences), generating new insights into health matters from individual as well as global perspectives on population health. The principal domains explored in Health and Society are hospitals, communities, medicine, social policies, medico-sanitary institutions, and health systems.

Previous titles in the *Health and Society* collection

Robert J. Flynn, Meagan Miller, Tessa Bell, Barbara Greenberg, and Cynthia Vincent, *Young People in Out-of-Home Care: Findings from the Ontario Looking After Children Project*, 2023.

Lloyd Hawkeye Robertson, *The Evolved Self: Mapping an Understanding of Who We Are*, 2020.

Sylvie Frigon, ed., *Dance: Confinement and Resilient Bodies / Danse : Enfermenent et corps résilients*, 2019.

Martin Rovers, Judith Malette, and Manal Guirguis-Younger, eds., *Touch in the Helping Professions: Research, Practice and Ethics*, 2018.

Serge Brochu, Natacha Brunelle, and Chantal Plourde, *Drugs and Crime: A Complex Relationship*. Third revised and expanded edition, 2018.

Marie Drolet, Pier Bouchard, and Jacinthe Savard, eds., *Accessibility and Active Offer: Health Care and Social Services in Linguistic Minority Communities*, 2017.

Isabelle Perreault and Marie Claude Thifault, eds., *Récits inachevés : Réflexions sur les défis de la recherche qualitative*, 2016.

Mamadou Barry and Hachimi Sanni Yaya, *Financement de la santé et efficacité de l'aide internationale*, 2015.

For a complete list of the University of Ottawa Press titles, please visit:
www.Press.uOttawa.ca

www.ingramcontent.com/pod-product-compliance
Lightning Source LLC
Chambersburg PA
CBHW070324270326
41926CB00017B/3758